# The Cleaning, Hygiene and Maintenance Handbook

# The Cleaning, Hygiene and Maintenance Handbook

Terence P. McLaughlin, B.Sc., A.R.I.C.

Prentice-Hall, Inc., Englewood Cliffs, N.J.

Prentice-Hall International, Inc., *London*
Prentice-Hall of Australia, Pty. Ltd., *Sydney*
Prentice-Hall of Canada, Ltd., *Toronto*
Prentice-Hall of India Private Ltd., *New Delhi*
Prentice-Hall of Japan, Inc., *Tokyo*

Original British edition published in 1969 by Business Books Limited, London. United States edition published in 1973 by Prentice-Hall, Inc.

The reader is advised to consult the Pure Food and Drug Act, as well as the nearest office of the Department of Labor, to determine if there is any regulation of the Occupational Safety and Health Act which may apply to the substances, devices, or procedures described herein.

This publication is designed to provide accurate and authoritative information in regard to the subject matter covered. It is sold with the understanding that the publisher is not engaged in rendering legal, accounting or other professional service. If legal advice or other expert assistance is required, the services of a competent professional person should be sought.

*... From the Declaration of Principles jointly adopted by a Committee of the American Bar Association and a Committee of Publishers and Associations.*

**Library of Congress Cataloging in Publication Data**

McLaughlin, Terence.
    The cleaning, hygiene and maintenance handbook.

    1. Industrial housekeeping. 2. Factory sanitation. I. Title. [DNLM: 1. Industrial medicine. WA 400 M161c 1973]
TS193. M3 1973       648'.5        72-14158
ISBN 0-13-136606-8

Printed in the United States of America

# About the Author

Terence McLaughlin, B.Sc., A.R.I.C., has long been concerned with various aspects of cleaning and detergency. Several years of basic research and product development have given him an insight into the scientific background of cleaning and surface treatment and a detailed knowledge of detergents and finishing agents.

As Development Manager and Director of a major detergent company, he has been responsible for the development and testing of cleaning and finishing products, liaison with machinery manufacturers, and advisory departments dealing with cleaning and hygiene problems. He now directs a consulting service, McLaughlin and Golding Project Developments, which offers advice on all cleaning matters.

Mr. McLaughlin has written on many aspects of cleaning, including chemical scouring and water treatment. He has also contributed extensively to books on cosmetic chemistry.

# A Word from the Author

Maintenance is often taken to imply only the business of dealing with repairs and replacements of plant, equipment, and buildings, whether on a scheduled plan or on an *ad hoc* basis, but there is another important side to it. All the features that go to make up an office or plant—floors, walls, rugs, furniture, kitchen equipment and so on—need repair or replacement at some time or other, but the length of time between repairs and replacement depends on a more unobtrusive kind of maintenance that goes on every day—using the right cleaning materials, applying the right finish, making sure that the grit is removed from a rug before it can cut the pile or removing a stain from a floor before it becomes permanent. There is an old proverb that says "one keep-clean is worth ten make-cleans," and it is certainly true that the conscientious cleaner can save, if not ten, at least some of the visits of the maintenance engineer.

Cleaning and maintenance on the day-to-day basis is not a glamorous side of industry, and rarely dramatic, except when some neglect causes a disaster, such as an outbreak of food poisoning, the spoiling of some valuable furniture, or the discovery by the company president that there is old lipstick on his coffee cup. The best cleaning and maintenance work goes on unobtrusively and usually unnoticed.

This often means, unfortunately, that the maintenance manager is not given the same scope to improve and modernize his methods as, say, the accountant or the salesman, and the same standards of productivity and efficiency may not be applied to his department. This is not solely because cleaning and maintenance is a service activity, and not a profit-making one: office management and catering are equally services, but a great deal of time and effort is spent in seeing that these activities are carried out with the greatest efficiency—and, more important, with the correct tools and materials.

The primary trouble is the belief among some senior members of management that cleaning, and its organization, is something that can be left to the janitor or a supervisor, and that it represents such a small item of expenditure that it would not pay to spend much time in reviewing the methods or materials used. This is a serious and expensive error. Not only are the costs of cleaning and maintenance a significant item in the budget of any company, but the results of the maintenance work have a profound effect, for good or ill, on the costs of repairs and replacements, staff-management relations, the health, safety, and productivity of staff, the safety of customers, in some cases, and the general image of the company projected to members of the public who visit company plant or offices. The cleanliness of the work environment has an enormous psychological effect on employees, partly because they tend to identify their working conditions with the management, and partly because a neat and tidy office or workshop encourages neat and conscientious work. Employees may listen politely when they are told about the good intentions of the management, but they will still draw their own conclusions from a dirty washroom or stained dishes.

The purpose of this book, then, is to help maintenance personnel do the best possible job, using the materials and machinery designed to do the job, at the lowest expenditure of time and money.

Terence P. McLaughlin

# Table of Contents

       Soap . Hard Soap . Toilet Soap Laundry Flakes .
       Soap Powders . Liquid Toilet Soap . Soft Soap

       Anionic Detergents . Biodegradability . Cationic
       Detergents . Nonionic Detergents . Amphoteric
       Detergents . Detergent Powders . Detergent Liquids
       . Scouring Powders

       Alcohol . Acetone . Gasoline . White Spirit

**Chapter Five: Tools and Machines** *(cont.)*

## PART II

Heavy-Duty Floorings . Concrete . Concrete Tiles
or Flags . Monolithic Concrete Paving . Metal-Clad
Flags . Granolithic . Asphalt Cement (Bituminous
Cement) . Latex Cement . Mastic Asphalt . Pitch-
mastic . Composition Blocks . Bricks and Other
Paving Materials . Unglazed Tiles . Ceramic Fully
Vitrified Tiles . Magnesite . Epoxy Resins . Polyester
Resins . Polyurethane Resins . End-Grain Wood
Blocks . Metal Anchor Plates and Metal Paving Tiles
. Jointing Compounds . Medium Duty Floorings .
Marble, Natural Stone . Terrazzo . Wood . Cork .
Linoleum . Rubber . Epoxy Resins, Polyester
Resins, Polyurethane Resins . Asphalt Tiles . Vinyl
Tiles

Concrete . Iron Stains . Copper Stains . Ink Stains .
Lubricating Oil . Fire Stains . Rotten Wood . Iodine
Stains . Urine Stains . Crayon Marks . Paint . Blood-
stains . Glazed Tiles . Wood, Cork, Linoleum . Coffee
and Tea Stains . Marking Ink . Magnesite . Vinyl
Tiles

**Chapter Ten: Kitchens** *(cont.)*

# List of Figures

# List of Plates

# one

# The Cost of Cleaning and Hygiene

The national expenditure on cleaning and cleaning materials is difficult to assess exactly, because many materials that can be used for cleaning have other uses besides, and therefore figure in several sets of statistics. Additionally, personnel employed for cleaning work may carry out other duties, and some will be classified in government reports as engaged in catering, repair and maintenance, and miscellaneous job descriptions. However, with one or two reasonable assumptions, a figure can be calculated.

Household expenditure in the United States on cleaning materials in 1968 was about $3.15 billion at retail values, and industrial expenditure about $800 million, making $3.95 billion in all. This bought, among other items, about 2,500,000 tons of soaps and detergents, plus polishes, sanitizers, hand cleansers, sweeping compounds, floor sealing materials, specialty cleansers, and so on. In these days the amount of cleaning labor paid for on the household market is relatively small, but in the industrial sector several analyses agree that labor cost is now about 70 per cent of the total cost of cleaning, while materials of all kinds only account for about 20 per cent (the balance is for cleaning machinery), so the total cost of industrial cleaning in 1968 was around $3.6 billion. The complete cleaning budget therefore appears as in Table 1.1.

| Table 1.1 The Cost of Cleaning | $ million |
|---|---|
| Household cleaning materials | 3,150 |
| Household cleaning labor (estimated) | 200 |
| Industrial cleaning materials | 800 |
| Industrial cleaning labor | 2,800 |
| Household machinery for cleaning | 800 |
| Industrial machinery for cleaning | 500 |
| Total | $8,250 million |

*17*

These figures do not include laundry machinery.

With such sums at stake, it is sensible to try to investigate whether the right products and machines are being bought, and whether they are used properly in the cleaners' hands. The materials represent a significant proportion of the gross national product, and the labor required costs only a little less than the materials, so even a small saving in cleaning costs could have an effect on the total economy. However, the main emphasis in the chapters that follow is not the making of marginal savings, but carrying out each cleaning operation with the best products and the best methods to meet the circumstances. The methods described are those that will contribute most towards the safe upkeep of premises and equipment, and towards the setting up of a hygienic and safe environment for workers and customers. Such a criterion of the best cleaning methods will contribute more to long-term savings than efforts to shave a cent off the price of a bucket of detergent, or to make do with one washing where two are really necessary. Fortunately, in most cases, the best methods of cleaning for the purposes of hygiene are also the quickest and easiest:

## CLEANING MATERIALS—USAGE

The amounts of various cleaning materials used in household and industrial cleaning give a good idea of the complexity of the market. Table 1.2 shows the estimated sales value of the most important types of product in 1967. The figures have been separated into household and industrial sales.

The percentage figures for industrial sales show a move towards specialized cleansers and finishes at the expense of the general-purpose liquids and powders. Where many housewives will make use of a conventional detergent powder for laundry, dishwashing, and general cleaning work, the industrial user has learned the advantages of buying products which are tailor-made for each specific purpose.

## BREAKDOWN OF COSTS

Surveys in the hotel trade have shown a fairly constant pattern of costs in large and small establishments, which can be expressed as in Table 1.3. These figures are based on housekeepers' costs collected by the American Hotel and Motel Association.

**Table 1.2 Sales Value of Cleaning Products in the United States, 1967**

| Product | Household sales ($ million) | Percentage | Industrial sales ($ million) | Percentage |
|---|---|---|---|---|
| Soaps, detergents | 1,047 | 34.9 | 210 | 28.0 |
| Waxes and finishes | 765 | 25.5 | 155 | 20.7 |
| Surface cleaners | 135 | 4.5 | 31.5 | 4.2 |
| Rug shampoos | 135 | 4.5 | 31.5 | 4.2 |
| Hand cleansers | 156 | 5.2 | 31.5 | 4.2 |
| Sanitizers | 216 | 7.2 | 40 | 5.3 |
| Aerosols | 234 | 7.8 | 95 | 12.7 |
| Toilet cleansers | 66 | 2.2 | 12 | 1.6 |
| Deodorant blocks | 9 | 0.3 | 3.75 | 0.5 |
| Insecticides | 78 | 2.6 | 64 | 8.5 |
| Sweeping compounds | 21 | 0.7 | 12 | 1.6 |
| Floor seals | 39 | 1.3 | 16 | 2.1 |
| Boiler compounds | 24 | 0.8 | 8 | 1.1 |
| Ice-melting compounds | 24 | 0.8 | 12 | 1.6 |
| Specialty cleansers | 45 | 1.5 | 24 | 3.2 |
| Miscellaneous | 6 | 0.2 | 3.75 | 0.5 |
| | 3,000 | 100.0 | 750.0 | 100.0 |

**Table 1.3 Percentage Costs of Cleaning Materials**

|                                                    | *Percentage* |
|----------------------------------------------------|--------------|
| Labor cost                                         | 70.00        |
| Soaps and detergents                               | 1.25         |
| Sanitizers and deodorizers                         | 1.33         |
| Floor finishes                                     | 1.00         |
| Mops, brooms etc.                                  | 3.25         |
| Other cleansers                                    | 2.25         |
| Remaining recurring items                          | 15.00        |
| Non-recurring items<br>(amortization of equipment) | 5.92         |
|                                                    | 100.00%      |

In other establishments, such as hospitals and factories, reliable surveys are hard to find, but of those that exist a constant pattern is the high proportion of labor cost, which seems to approach 70 per cent. Otherwise the pattern is variable. Hospitals spend a greater proportion on actual cleaning agents than factories, and this probably reflects the demand for such materials as really effective sanitizers and similar hygiene promoters in the hospitals.

Of all these costs, it is generally agreed that the most costly area of maintenance is the floor. This is the part of any building that receives the most wear and is subjected to the worst treatment, especially in bad weather. The maintenance problems of the floor may be appreciated from the details in Chapter Six. A summary of various partial surveys of the maintenance costs of various types of buildings suggests the following rough breakdown of costs:

**Table 1.4 Distribution of Costs in Building Maintenance**

|                                  | *Percentage* |
|----------------------------------|--------------|
| Floors                           | 40           |
| Equipment and machinery cleaning | 24           |
| Walls, woodwork                  | 16           |
| Ceilings                         | 8            |
| Windows and skylights            | 7            |
| Lighting fixtures                | 5            |
|                                  | 100%         |

This means, among other things, that we spend about $1.6 billion per year on keeping floors clean, and about half of this enormous sum is spent by industrial users.

## CHOICE OF MATERIALS

The chapters that follow detail cleaning materials, germicidal materials, and cleaning tools and machines, before passing on to the detailed study of various cleaning jobs. The object of this introductory chapter is to highlight the main principles which direct the choice of this or that material or machine for a given purpose. The buyer who deals with cleaning materials is not usually kept short of product information from the manufacturers of detergents or machines, but he may well be wary about accepting all this information as the whole story. While reputable manufacturers or their salesmen will not deceive a customer, they may well tend to inflate the value of their own wares a little; so that a detergent that is, at most, merely acceptable for a certain cleaning task is presented as if it were specially formulated for the job, and a machine that can, with a struggle, perform adequately, is described as ideal for the circumstances.

In addition, as the detergent companies in particular are usually provided with highly trained technical personnel, who *can* be extremely helpful to a customer, there is a risk that the buyer who is not technically qualified may be "blinded with science" by the salesman or technical service man. The following chapters are intended to describe not only the products and machines, but also the scientific jargon that surrounds them, so that the buyer of cleaning products or equipment can profit better from the genuinely helpful technical man, and avoid being confused by the other kind.

# PART I

# Cleaning Materials and Equipment

# two

# Cleaning Products

The greater part of maintenance work is concerned with the removal of dirt, and the choice of the best cleaning materials for each job is the maintenance manager's most important buying decision. The actual cost of soaps, detergents, polishes and so on may be only about 5 per cent of the total cost of maintenance, but the use of unsuitable products will certainly lead to a waste of time—and time, in terms of labor cost, is the most expensive item in any cleaning program.

Unfortunately, the wide range of available soaps, detergents, polishes, sanitizers, and other cleaning products, and the often conflicting claims of the manufacturers, make the choice more difficult. It would be impossible in the compass of this book to describe all the available types of cleaning material in detail, but a few general principles may be laid down to assist in the selection of the most suitable product for each purpose.

Removal of solid dirt particles usually presents no great problems: cotton and other cellulosic fibers tend to hold on to dirt by electrical forces, but in most cases solid dry dirt would come away very easily. However, dirt is usually mixed with greasy or oily materials, and these represent the real problem. The greasy layer may be derived from the human body, as on clothes; or from toiletries such as hair cream and cosmetics; from food preparation, serving, and eating; from vehicle exhausts, machinery and fuel; on floors it may be associated with rubber from shoes and the mixture of tire rubber, oil and tar that is tracked in from the streets. The detergent chemist, whose chief opponent is grease, finds it present on almost every conceivable surface.

All oils and fats, whether animal, vegetable, mineral, or synthetic, owe their characteristic "oily" properties–slipperiness, easy softening under pressure or heat, incompatibility with water, and so on–to a chemical grouping consisting of long chains of carbon atoms surrounded by hydrogen atoms:

$$
\begin{array}{ccccccc}
H & H & H & H & H & H & H \\
| & | & | & | & | & | & | \\
H-C-&C-&C-&C-&C-&C-&C- \\
| & | & | & | & | & | & | \\
H & H & H & H & H & H & H
\end{array}
$$

usually shortened to $CH_3CH_2CH_2CH_2CH_2CH_2CH_2-$ or $C_7H_{15}$ for convenience and brevity. The number of carbon atoms can vary enormously–very light mineral oil products such as gasoline may contain only five, six, or seven (as in the example above); heavy waxes may contain a hundred or more. Whatever the size of the group, however, it is called a *hydrocarbon* group. Most mineral oils are composed entirely of such hydrocarbon groups, while animal and vegetable oils contain a very high proportion of them.

As is well known, water by itself is of very little use in removing oils and fats from surfaces because it will not "wet" a surface covered with oil, whereas most materials containing hydrocarbon groups will mix quite easily with other hydrocarbon materials–oil or gasoline will penetrate and soften a hard wax, or a solid fat like tallow, very easily. Many solvents contain hydrocarbon groups, and to this they owe their powers of grease removal. However, solvents are not suitable for many cleaning operations because of fire or health hazards, apart from the cost, and it is necessary therefore to invent some way of inducing the hydrocarbon groups to disperse in water. This is the principle underlying all the technology of soaps and detergents.

Soaps and detergents contain hydrocarbon groups combined with other chemical groupings that make the whole substance water-soluble. Like tame elephants mixing with wild ones and helping to control them, the hydrocarbon groups of the detergent mix with the hydrocarbon groups of the grease or oil which we are trying to remove, and the water-soluble groups then carry the whole of the oily hydrocarbon material into the water. This is shown diagrammatically in Figure 2.1, where the wavy lines represent hydrocarbon groups, and the black circles water-soluble groups.

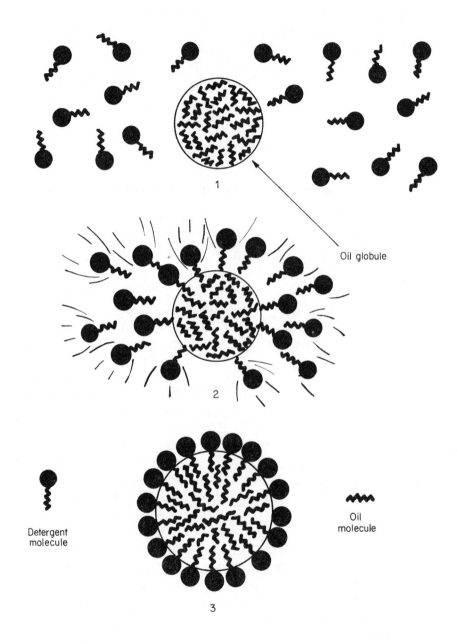

Figure 2.1

(1) Oil globule surrounded by detergent molecules. (2) Detergent molecules surrounding oil globule. (3) Oil globule is surrounded by the water-soluble portions of the detergent molecules.

For cleaning surfaces, there is another requirement of the detergent. The grease on a surface is usually stuck firmly to it, and is not easily detached by water, even with the aid of a detergent material. To remove the grease quickly and efficiently, the detergent must have a stronger affinity for the surface than the grease has. If this criterion is satisfied, detergent solution can creep between the grease and the surface and "pry off" the grease layer. Figure 2.2 illustrates this: a layer of grease is lifted up at one end, and eventually rolls into spherical drops which are taken up by the detergent solution. Photomicrographs have shown this process actually going on.

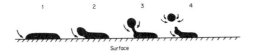

Figure 2.2

(1) Oily dirt lying on a surface. (2) Detergent solution penetrates under one end. (3) Portion of oil is almost surrounded by detergent. (4) Oil lifted away as oil globule and next section of the oily dirt is penetrated by detergent.

Materials used for cleaning, in fact, must have the ability to surround and suspend oily particles—*emulsifying action*—and the ability to attach to a surface more strongly than the grease—*wetting action*. Their efficiency as cleansers is a combination of the two actions. For certain specialized purposes there are requirements for one or the other property alone, but a cleanser needs both. Fortunately for the chemist who designs detergents, many of the water-soluble groups that impart wetting action also impart emulsifying action, and vice versa.

## TYPES OF DETERGENT

Detergents (and, to the chemist, soap is a type of detergent) thus consist of two groups fastened together, the hydrocarbon group and the water-soluble group, and as variations are possible in both, a very large number of different detergents can be made. In practice, the hydrocarbon groups are taken from available fatty materials with two main criteria— low cost and chemical suitability for attaching a water-soluble group. Some very cheap sources of hydrocarbon, like kerosene, are difficult to combine chemically with suitable water-soluble groups, while the more expensive animal and vegetable oils and fats are easy to convert. They are so easy to make into a cleansing substance, in fact, that the process has been known for centuries, and we call the product *soap*.

SOAP

Animal and vegetable fats and oils consist almost entirely of *glycerides,* or compounds of fatty acids, which are sources of hydrocarbon material, with glycerin. Soaps are manufactured by treating the glycerides with the alkalis sodium or potassium hydroxide; the basic equation of the process is as follows:

fat (= fatty acid + glycerin) + sodium hydroxide = soap + glycerin.

The glycerin is almost always recovered from the soap and sold separately as a valuable by-product. The state of the glycerin market, and especially the price of synthetic glycerin, thus has an effect on the basic price of soap.

Soaps as a class are generally good cleansers, but there are distinctions which can be made within the class, according to the type of fat or oil used for manufacturing the soap. Soap makers recognize three main types of starting material: hard fats (such as tallow or palm oil), soft oils (such as whale oil or peanut oil), and nut oils, mainly coconut and palm kernel fat; these differ in their properties because of the different proportions of various glycerides which they contain. Hard fats produce a soap that is hard in texture, not very soluble in cold water, slow to lather, but with thick and persistent suds once these have been worked up. It is, however, an excellent cleansing agent with first-class detergency and dirt-suspending properties, and keeps well without any tendency to become rancid. Soft oils produce a soap that is soft in texture, easily soluble even in cold water, quick to lather (though the suds may collapse quickly), fairly good as a detergent but inclined to go rancid and deteriorate in color and odor. Nut oils produce a soap that is hard but easily soluble in water, quick to lather with an open foam consisting of large bubbles, but very poor as a cleansing agent. Nut oils are generally more expensive than the other materials.

The soap maker uses his knowledge of these properties to the best advantage, mixing the oils and fats to make a soap suitable for each job. A commercial laundry soap, for instance, to be used at high temperatures and needing the very best possible detergency for economic reasons, will be made from hard fats almost entirely, and tallow is usually selected. Such a soap will not dissolve or lather easily except near the boiling point, but that is how the launderer will use it. By contrast, a soap to be used for washing the hands and face, and therefore in lukewarm water, must dissolve and lather much more easily; it must also be hard in consistency, otherwise the bar will be wasteful. Nut oil soaps alone would be suitable from the point of view of suds and consistency, but they are expensive and also rather irritating to the skin, so the soap maker uses a mixture of soaps of hard fat with enough nut oil soap to give the required quick lather: usually 80 per cent tallow and 20 per cent coconut oil.

Soaps for technical industrial use, especially if they are intended for mixing with other ingredients, need not be of such good color and odor as toilet soap, so the manufacturer can use the cheaper soft oils; the so-called *acid oils* extracted during the refining of edible oil are often used in this way. Soap makers know that the same final mixture of soaps can be achieved by using different proportions of the complex mixtures of glycerides in natural fats and oils (the mixture may vary according to the source, the season, the weather in which vegetable fats were produced, the method of extraction, and so on), and they calculate their formulae to give the required result at the lowest price (for, again, the prices of the various fats and oils will vary greatly at different periods, if there are droughts, or poor crops, or other effects on the yield of oil). Some manufacturers even use computers to keep their product composition constant while allowing for variations in the composition and price of the raw materials.

Apart from the variations in fatty acid composition, the soap may vary in another respect—moisture content. Soap making is a process carried out in solution, and soap hangs on to its moisture tenaciously. In fact, perfectly dry soap, free of all moisture, would be something of a laboratory curiosity. Soap as first produced contains about 32 per cent water, and in this condition it can be melted fairly easily and processed as a hot viscous liquid. If this liquid is allowed to cool, it becomes *hard soap,* the simplest soap product, familiar as bars of kitchen or "scrubbing" soap. This commodity is still sold, but in steadily diminishing amounts, and no doubt the next ten years or so will see its complete disappearance. The old method of making hard soap bars was to fill a large container, the "frame," with melted soap, then allow this to set and cut it into bars. Now the soap is shaped into a long continuous bar in a "plodder" and cut into appropriate lengths.

For toilet soap use, hard soap tends to wear away too quickly and is also rather coarse in texture. Toilet soaps are therefore milled several times to break up any crystalline soap that might coarsen the texture, and dried to about 16 per cent moisture.

For soap flakes and chips, the product must be dried even further as otherwise the flakes will stick together, and 91 per cent soap is the usual level. For certain specialized purposes soap is made in the form of a pure powder, with up to 98 per cent soap and less than 2 per cent moisture, but this requires prolonged drying and stoving, which is an expensive process.

As well as these products containing only soap and moisture, essentially, there are many mixtures. For general cleaning purposes soap may be mixed with other materials which extend its cleaning action, usually alkalis, which have themselves some power of grease removal. The "soap powders" that are sold for dishwashing, general cleaning and laundering are mixtures of soap and soda ash—dried sodium carbonate, which is "washing soda" in the crystalline form. Those intended especially for laundry use also contain other ingredients which will be considered later.

The maintenance manager who buys soap is thus buying a complex commodity; the soap characteristics may vary, the moisture content may vary, other additives may or may not be present. Fortunately standards have been laid down for many of these variables, and analysts have invented simple tests to ascertain the quality of the soap in terms of these variables. First, the type of fat or oil used as the raw material can be ascertained by gas-liquid chromatography (G.L.C.) analysis. This method depends on the fact that every fat or oil contains a mixture of hydrocarbon chains of different lengths, some with a few carbon atoms linked together, others with many. In general, hard fats contain long hydrocarbon groups, with 16-18 carbon atoms in the majority and a small quantity of shorter (10-14 carbon atoms) material. Nut oils contain shorter hydrocarbon groups, with 10-14 carbon atoms. Soft oils contain a large proportion of *oleic acid,* which has 18 carbon atoms but with a different type of chemical structure. The G.L.C. apparatus measures directly the proportions of each type of hydrocarbon group present in a fat, a mixture of fats, or the soap made from them, and by comparison with known materials it is usually possible to deduce the make-up of any sample. Large manufacturers with reasonable laboratory facilities are always ready to provide G.L.C. standards when the customer needs a very accurate specification of quality.

For many purposes, the accuracy of the G.L.C. test is far greater than is necessary; differences in the G.L.C. analysis may not give rise to any detectable differences in the soap itself. In such cases there is a rough and ready test: the analyst splits the soap into its fatty acids and measures the melting point of the mixture; this is known in the jargon of the trade as the *titer.* High titers, around 95°-120°F, correspond to hard fats, lower ones to nut oils, and very low ones to soft oils. Mixtures of fats will give intermediate titer figures.

The *soap content* of a sample, as distinct from the moisture or other ingredients, is measured by finding the proportion of fatty acid and calculating from this the amount of soap. Thus a typical soap flake or chip may be analyzed and found to contain 84 per cent fatty acid, or a soap powder may contain 20 per cent; the corresponding soap contents (expressed as water-free or *anhydrous* soap) will be 91 per cent and 21.7 per cent respectively. If the manufacturers quote fatty acid contents only—an archaic practice arising from analysts' convenience—it is usually sufficient to use the equation:

$$(\text{fatty acid per cent}) \times 13/12 = \text{soap per cent}$$

Because of the moisture content of all types of soap, there exists a possibility that some of this moisture will dry out on storage: obviously hard and toilet soaps, which contain substantial amounts of water, are most likely to lose it. The customer should remember in this case that only *moisture* is being lost, not soap. A box of 100 pounds of soap at 82.8 per cent anhydrous soap contains about 15 pounds of water and 82.8 pounds of anhydrous soap. If the soap dries out to, say, 96 pounds during storage, there are still 82.8 pounds of soap. The only loss is four pounds of water. This fact must be remembered when marked packs of soap products do not appear to contain the full weight marked: manufacturers of cheese and other moisture-containing commodities have similar difficulties, but fortunately their goods are not stored as long as soap.

As soaps are made with sodium hydroxide, a caustic alkali, it is obviously important that as little as possible of the unchanged alkali should be left in the product. It might be thought safer to use a slight surplus of fat or fatty acid to neutralize all the alkali with certainty, but unfortunately it is found in practice that this causes the soap to turn rancid very quickly. The soap maker therefore finishes off the soap with a very small and carefully controlled amount of surplus alkali, quite insufficient to cause any harm to the skin. Sodium carbonate, a milder alkali, may also be present, and slightly larger quantities of this can be tolerated. Soap analysts therefore recognize two types of alkali in soap, *carbonate alkali* and *caustic alkali*. The latter is obviously more important as a potential hazard, and the term "free alkali" which is often given in specifications usually means caustic alkali. Both types are usually quoted as sodium hydroxide, NaOH.

Two other characteristics of soap which are mentioned in analytical tests and specifications may be reviewed briefly. *Rosin content* is sometimes quoted, as a maximum permitted proportion. This provision dates from the days, now long ago, when rosin was cheaper than fat and was used as a diluting agent. It is hardly used at all now except in specialized soaps, mainly because today it costs more than fat. *Chloride content* in soap arises from brine used during manufacture. Excessive chloride can do no harm to the user, but may make soap tablets crack or show a slight "bloom" on the surface.

We can now summarize the various types of soap product by giving, for each type, suitable standards that the buyer ought to expect from his suppliers. A.S.T.M. standards, where they exist, represent a good *minimum* standard, but in most cases the products of reputable manufacturers will be better than this minimum.

### Hard Soap

If this commodity is required for laundry work, scrubbing, or as a cheap substitute for toilet soap, it should be firm, smooth, mild in odor, pale or clear in color (not "muddy" looking), and show no cracks or crystalline patches. Such soap can be supplied with an anhydrous soap content of 65-68 per cent, free (caustic) alkali as NaOH less than 0.2 per cent, free acid (as oleic acid) less than 0.5 per cent, chloride as sodium chloride less than 1.0 per cent. The A.S.T.M. standard D497-52 (reapproved 1967) for laundry bar soap may be used for a minimum standard, but it allows a very low level of anhydrous soap (52 per cent minimum) and the existing standard permits a maximum of 0.5 per cent free alkali. There was, however, a recommendation to lower this level in the 1968 A.S.T.M. standards.

### Toilet Soap

Toilet soap bars should be smooth and have no detectable odor apart from the added perfume. The anhydrous soap content should be at least 80 per cent, with no rosin in the fatty matter. As such soap is specifically for use on the skin, free caustic alkali should not be more than 0.02 per cent, and total caustic and carbonate alkali not more than 0.1 per cent, both as NaOH. Rosin acids and sugar (sometimes added to improve the texture) should not be included in good-quality toilet soap. The chloride content should be less than 0.5 per cent.

Some toilet soaps contain a small amount of fatty material such as petroleum jelly or mineral oil; this is known as *super-fatting*. There is no evidence that such treatment produces any other effect than a slight thickening of the lather of the soap; claims that such simple means "feed the skin" or otherwise beautify the user are quite unfounded. Other additives likely to be found are, of course, perfume, and whitening agents such as titanium dioxide. Toilet soap which has been milled extensively—a process which improves the texture—tends to look slightly translucent, and this makes a white soap look rather dull or even dirty in some lights. Titanium dioxide is therefore added to opaque the bars.

In the domestic market there is a recent tendency to introduce a modified form of toilet soap that contains a large proportion of unneutralized fatty acid, deliberately added in the milling stages. Such soap is claimed to have beneficial effects on the skin; certainly the texture of the soap and the type of lather is much improved. Soap made in this way is more expensive than the traditional toilet soap. The standards given above would apply to such bars.

Floating soap is ordinary toilet soap that has been foamed up, or made with a cavity, so that the total weight of the bar is less than that of the same volume of water. There is an A.S.T.M. standard, D499-48 (reapproved 1967) for such soap; the maximum levels for free alkali (0.1 per cent), rosin acids (nil) and similar characteristics are similar to the standards given above; the anhydrous soap level can, however, be as low as 62.0 per cent.

## Laundry Flakes

A special variety of soap is made in flake form for laundering purposes, an operation which comes under the responsibilities of many maintenance managers. The greater part of all laundering work, whether in commercial laundries, industry or hospitals, is concerned with white work—table linen, bed linen, white coats and overalls, etc.—which is best washed at a high temperature. The soap for such work should therefore be suitable for high levels of detergency at the boiling point or near it, and its performance at low temperatures is not so important. For the reasons stated earlier such a soap is best made from hard fats, and a good grade of tallow is almost universally used as the basis for laundry soap.

The soap is often introduced into the washing machines in the form of a solution: a stock solution of 2½ per cent or 5 per cent is made up, and this is introduced into the machines by volume, in most cases by automatic controls.

For the best effects, the soap should be supplemented by sodium carboxymethylcellulose (SCMC), a synthetic gum. SCMC has the very useful property, for the launderer, that it suspends dirt particles which have been removed from the soiled articles and keeps the dirt in suspension throughout the wash and rinse stages. This prevents the dirt from redepositing on the fabrics—a process that happens all to easily in the absence of SCMC, especially when the wash water is being drained off.

Extra soap will have the same "soil-suspending" action, but SCMC is more economical. SCMC at about 4 per cent of the actual weight of soap gives the best results; less may mean some redeposition of soiling matter, but more will mean waste. Most manufacturers of laundry soaps will supply flakes containing the correct proportion of SCMC, but it can also be purchased direct and added by the user to the stock solution.

Laundry soaps should also be used in conjunction with a suitable optical brightener. Optical brighteners, or fluorescent agents as they are sometimes called, are the modern successors to the old "laundry bluing." It is well known that, to the human eye, a bluish white appears "whiter" than a yellowish white, even though the two surfaces may reflect exactly the same quantity of light. If white washing is treated with a blue agent, such as ultramarine, the slight yellow color which is natural to cotton goods is made more blue, but at the expense of some of the reflected light—yellowish white has in fact been made bluish *gray*. The newer optical brighteners solve this problem by using the invisible ultraviolet light and converting this into visible blue light, thus adding to the total amount of reflected light from the washed articles and simultaneously making it bluer. This is the basis for claims by the manufacturers of washing powders that their products *brighten* washing.

Optical brighteners are dyestuffs, though of a peculiar kind, and like all dyestuffs they will not "take" easily on a greasy surface. It is therefore very important that laundry work should be thoroughly washed in the conventional way before the optical brighteners are absorbed. Otherwise, the optical brightener will be heavily absorbed on the clean parts of the work but greasy parts will not be brightened at all, and this will emphasize the contrast between clean and dirty areas. Pillow cases, which tend to become greasy in the center and remain clean at the edges, are particularly subject to this "picture frame" effect with optical brighteners unless they are really well washed; if they are not they come out of the tub with blued edges and yellow centers.

Most white fabrics are now treated with optical brighteners during manufacture, so the use of brighteners in laundering becomes necessary even if only to keep up the original appearance. Optical brighteners can be added by the user, but most laundry soap manufacturers can offer a flake complete with brightener already blended; this may cost more in terms of raw materials, but it will probably save labor costs.

Laundry flakes containing SCMC and optical brightener must, of course, have a somewhat lower soap content to allow for the other ingredients. The SCMC itself tends to stiffen up the soap and makes flaking more difficult. An acceptable level is around 80 per cent anhydrous soap with 3.2 per cent SCMC and optical brightener.

1749052

## Soap Powders

Alkalis such as sodium carbonate have a cleaning effect because they react with grease, particularly grease that has been aged in soiled fabrics, to produce a water-soluble soap. There are limits to this action, of course—alkalis have very little effect on mineral oil, for instance—but the addition of alkali to soap was developed as an economy measure many years ago. Such powders usually contain soap blended with sodium carbonate (the anhydrous material, soda ash, not the hydrated washing soda which tends to make powders cake badly). SCMC and fluorescent agents may also be added. In general, such powders have been outmoded by powders based on synthetic detergents.

For use in soft water, laundry powders are available in which tallow soap is blended with sodium carbonate, SCMC, and optical brighteners. These are very useful for concerns which have a small amount of laundry work to carry out—not enough to justify the installation of expensive stock solution plant.

A.S.T.M. standards give four types of soap powder for such laundry work, varying only in the type of soap used (this is adapted to the temperature of the wash). In general these powders should have a minimum of 50 per cent anhydrous soap (with no rosin in the fats), a total of 40 per cent alkali maximum (this includes alkali derived from the soap itself and that added deliberately), and a moisture content less than 16 per cent. The powders are designated as Type A (titer around 78° F), Type B (titer 78° - 85° F), Type C (titer over 85° F—i.e. high-temperature washing powder), and Type D, for which no titer limits are given. (Standard D533-44, reapproved 1967).

There is also a general-purpose powder (standard D 534-42, reapproved 1967) with anhydrous soap at a minimum of 15 per cent and alkali measured as sodium carbonate anhydrous at a minimum of 30 per cent.

## Liquid Toilet Soap

So far, all the soaps we have considered have been made from fats and sodium hydroxide. If the more expensive alkali, potassium hydroxide, is used, the soaps produced are very much more soluble in water, and can therefore be used in solution at concentrations up to about 25-30 per cent. This property is exploited for the production of liquid soaps that can be used in dispensers in washrooms. The liquid form of the product allows for economy in use and prevention of the pilfering that often takes place with soap bars.

Traditional liquid soaps are made from coconut or palm kernel fat, which give a clear, pale solution with a pleasant smell of the nuts from which the oil is extracted. However, such soaps are rather irritating to the skin, and should certainly not be used for washing the face. Many women in particular find this irritant effect so great that they will not use such soaps even on the hands. Other liquid soaps are made from cheap soft oils, such as partially hardened fish and whale oils or similar by-products of the margarine industry. These soaps are less irritating, but are darker in color and tend to have an unpleasant odor that persists on the hands for as much as an hour or two after washing.

It is possible to make liquid soaps with the same kind of fat charge as ordinary solid toilet soap (i.e. 80 per cent tallow and 20 per cent coconut or palm kernel fat), but these soap solutions are usually rather hazy, especially at low temperatures. However, such soap is very much milder on the skin than the nut oil soap, and has very little odor. The haziness can be concealed in part by making the product into an opaque cream.

The A.S.T.M. standard for liquid toilet soap (D799-62) deals with two types: Type A contains 15 per cent anhydrous potassium soap, and Type B 35 per cent anhydrous soap. The latter product would normally require alcohol or some similar material added to keep the soap in solution in cold weather. Total caustic alkali should not exceed 0.02 per cent in a good quality soap for the skin; some manufacturers add potassium carbonate to clarify the soap, but this is also quite alkaline and not to be recommended. Buyers should make sure that the soaps offered do not deposit solid matter at low temperatures, say 5° C, as otherwise they will tend to clog dispensers during the winter.

### Soft Soap

This is also a potassium soap, at a higher concentration than liquid soap. It was once used for cleaning, but is now virtually replaced by synthetic detergents. Small amounts of soft soap are made for applications where the jelly-like consistency is the most important feature—lubrication, etc.

## SYNTHETIC DETERGENTS

The greatest objection to soap products for cleansing is their behavior in hard water. In the presence of the dissolved calcium and magnesium salts that water picks up during its passage through the ground and over river beds, soap forms fatty acid salts of calcium and magnesium, and these "lime soaps," as they are loosely called, form an insoluble greasy scum on the surface of the water and curds under it. Not only does this use up soap that should have been active for cleansing, but the scum itself attaches to fibers, and the resulting mess may be very difficult to remove. On hard surfaces, such as tiled floors, the slippery lime soap may be a very real safety hazard, and soap should be avoided on such floors for this reason. Soaps are quite good cleansers in really soft water, but even a slight degree of hardness detracts from their performance.

Early in the nineteenth century it was discovered that olive and castor oils, treated with sulfuric acid, yielded a soapy material. The castor oil product soon found a use in dispersing the red dyestuff Turkey Red, much used in carpets, and was therefore called Turkey Red Oil. These *sulfated* compounds did not lather, but they were good emulsifiers and seemed to be almost unaffected by hard water. Later workers developed the process by using less expensive sources of fatty matter. During the 1920-1939 period, the Shell Petroleum Company in particular did much valuable work on detergents made from petroleum oils and sulfuric acid, and the shortage of natural fats in Germany during the 1939-45 war encouraged a vast increase in this research, particularly in Germany. These early products had certain disadvantages, but they shared one important property—they were all almost as effective in hard water as in soft.

Since this period, the detergent industry has mushroomed; there are now many thousands of synthetic detergents available on the market. However, most of these have very specialized uses, and the products of interest for normal cleansing and allied purposes can be limited to a few main types.

## Anionic Detergents

The classification of synthetic detergents is normally made by chemical type—anionic, cationic, nonionic, and amphoteric. These distinctions are of value to chemists who wish to compound mixtures of these detergents with one another or with other chemicals, but they have little value for the user except as names. It is sufficient to know that anionic and cationic detergents are of opposite chemical types and cannot be mixed without almost totally destroying one another's cleansing properties, while the nonionic and amphoteric detergents are more or less "neutral" and can be mixed with the others at will.

In terms of tonnage produced, the most important type of synthetic detergent is a group known variously as alkyl benzene sulfonates, alkyl aryl sulfonates, dodecyl benzene sulfonates or simply *DOBS*. This type is the basis of most household detergents, both powder and liquid. As with soaps, the fatty part of the molecule can be altered to give different properties, and at present there are two or three different *DOBS,* some being more soluble than the others and therefore used for liquid detergents, and others giving drier and crisper powders. Minor variations on these types are available, but the choice is limited because of the large capital plant needed to produce the raw materials.

The alkyl benzene sulfonates, as a class, are good detergents, with excellent foaming characteristics; they are not particularly good suspending agents for dirt and grease in themselves, but they can be blended with other materials to improve this action. These blends will be discussed later.

Alkyl benzene sulfonates, when entirely free from water, tend to be sticky or waxy solids and are not suitable for sale in the solid forms familiar with soap products. They are sold either as solutions in water or in a mixture with other powdered ingredients.

*Alkyl sulfates* or alcohol sulfates are a class of anionic detergent made by treating fatty alcohols, derived from natural fats and oils, with sulfuric acid or its compounds. They are used largely for hair shampoos and similar toiletries, as they are particularly mild in their effects. However, other uses of this class of detergent include:

1. Rug shampoos of the dry foam type, which are discussed in detail in Chapter Eight.
2. General detergents, where it is particularly important that all residues of detergent material shall be decomposed in effluent treatment.

The rug cleaner types are usually *lauryl sulfates,* derived from coconut oil, and the general detergents are usually *tallow alcohol sulfates,* derived from hard fats. The latter have first-class detergent properties for fabrics, etc., and are broken down completely during normal sewage treatment. They could, if produced on a large enough scale, be competitive in cost with the alkyl benzene sulfonates.

*Alkyl isethionates* are a type of anionic detergent mainly of importance for the production of synthetic toilet bars, intended to replace toilet soaps. They are not economically competitive with alkyl benzene sulfonates for ordinary purposes, but are very much milder in their action on the skin, the main concern in choosing a detergent for personal washing. Other anionic detergents which also have some importance in this field are: *alkyl glyceryl ether sulfates, sulfonated fatty acids* and *sulfated fatty acid monoglycerides.*

*Sulfated fatty ethers* and *amides* are developments from some of the nonionic detergents which are considered in a later section. They are anionic detergents of particularly high solubility and lathering power, and therefore find extensive use in the formulation of liquid detergents for dishwashing, etc., especially for the domestic market where the advertisers' ideal liquid gives voluminous lather with only a few drops of product in a sink full of water. The actual detergency of the two types is not superior to that of the alkyl benzene sulfonates.

## Biodegradability

One problem which has been introduced by the extensive use of synthetic detergents in household and industrial products in place of soap is the difficulty of removing residues of the newer materials from effluent. Soap is broken down entirely by bacteria in sewage treatment plants, forming either insoluble fat or even less embarrassing residues, and if any soap actually gets through to the rivers it is soon destroyed in the same way. The older types of alkyl benzene sulfonate were by no means so easy to decompose, and about 50 per cent of the residues might be found unchanged after months or even years of exposure to natural forces. They were, as water treatment specialists put it, not *biodegradable* or *biologically soft*. In the late 1940's and early 1950's the problem was becoming so acute that large banks of foam were forming on rivers at points of high agitation, such as dams and falls, and sewage plants operating on the activated sludge principle, where air is forced through the effluent, found that the detergent residues caused a serious foaming problem which was both an inconvenience and a health hazard. In rural areas, there were complaints of foaming water coming from the faucets; this was caused by detergent draining back from drainage systems into the water supply.

The solution was eventually found in new types of alkyl benzene sulfonates, which are now almost universally used. These detergents are at least 85 per cent decomposed in sewage treatment. A higher standard seems necessary, especially in highly populated areas where water has to be used several times during its flow in the rivers, but the situation is much improved.

## Cationic Detergents

This class of detergent, apart from specialized exceptions, is made by reacting fatty material with ammonium compounds as the water-soluble group, and they are often called by the chemists' name, *quaternary ammonium compounds* or *QAC*'s. They are usually poor in cleansing power and indifferent in lather, but they make up for these deficiencies by possessing two great advantages over the anionic detergents: QAC's are particularly mild in the action on textiles, and they are in fact used as the main ingredients in the "conditioners" and softeners used to restore the softness and smoothness to wool and other fibers after normal washing. QAC's can in some circumstances be used to wash textiles by themselves, but their cost and poor detergency tend to make it more economical to wash the fabrics with a conventional anionic detergent and then use the cationic one as a rinse.

The other advantage possessed by QAC's is that most of them have a marked germicidal effect. This appears to be a function of their effect on surfaces, as their germicidal action can be traced to an interference with the proper working of the cell wall of bacteria. Whatever the mechanism, QAC's are an extremely useful aid to bacteriological hygiene, and they will be considered in this role in the next chapter.

## Nonionic Detergents

These are detergents that are made from the normal sources of fatty matter (natural fats and oils, petroleum products, and so on), but these are made to react with various *non-ionizing* water-soluble groups that convert them into detergents. The most important nonionic detergents are those derived from fatty materials and *ethylene oxide,* a very reactive gas with the power of combining with many other substances, and also of forming a *polymer chain* of several molecules of ethylene oxide itself. The polymer is called polyethylene glycol, and like its simplest form, ethylene glycol (used widely as anti-freeze), is very soluble in water. The detergents made by connecting this polymer of ethylene oxide with fatty materials are called variously *polyoxyethylene compounds, polyethylene glycol compounds, alkyl phenol polyoxyethylene adducts,* and so on, according to type and the personal preferences of the writer, and nomenclature can be very confusing. In general, however, it is safe to say that most of the detergents with the names *polyoxyethylene* or *polyethylene glycol* in their descriptions are nonionic.

Nonionic detergents, in general, are characterized by poor foaming power, but they are very good emulsifiers and detergents, with particular powers of removing mineral oil soiling. The most common types are made from alkyl phenols and ethylene oxide.

Detergents of this type are quite unsuitable for use in solid products, as even the 100 per cent product is quite fluid. They are therefore used invariably as liquid detergents. For many purposes they are quite satisfactory on their own, but their low lathering characteristic may be a disadvantage, not only from the psychological point of view, but also because the unskilled user may have no indication of the degree of exhaustion of a wash liquid. They are therefore often blended with anionic detergents which produce a satisfactory degree of lather. In any case the combination is a good one, because nonionic detergents are usually more expensive than anionic ones, especially of the DOBS type.

Another type of nonionic detergent is the group of *alkanolamides* or *alkylolamides* (the names are interchangeable) which are made from fatty acids and amines. These materials are not very effective detergents on their own, but when blended with DOBS anionic detergents they have several valuable properties. They stabilize the foam, they increase the solubility of the main detergent, and they increase the suspending action for dirt. They are therefore used as lather stabilizers in powder detergents, and solubilizing agents and lather stabilizers in liquid detergents.

## Amphoteric Detergents

These combine some of the properties of anionic and cationic detergents: they are usually cationic in character in acid solutions and anionic in alkaline solutions. They are used mainly in applications where their germicidal action, in the cationic form, can be exploited.

## Detergent Powders

The use of synthetic detergents in cleansing agents became familiar in the 1940's, when powders for domestic use were first introduced. An enormous tonnage of such products is now made—over two million tons per annum in the United States alone. The scale of the operation is very important economically, as the plant used for manufacturing these powders is an extremely large capital outlay, and only by the greatest degree of mass production can it operate efficiently. This large concentration of capital in the plant has had two important effects. The detergent powder industry is in the hands of a very few large manufacturers, of which the largest are Procter and Gamble, Colgate, and Lever Brothers, on a worldwide basis, and the formulations tend to be standardized for long periods without major changes because every change of formula means an expensive period of modification on the plant.

It is possible, for this reason, to describe a typical detergent powder formulation which is not far removed from the main products of the major suppliers. This is probably the best way to explain the various ingredients that are used in such powders, and their role in the performance of the product.

A typical detergent powder for general application, therefore, would have a formula something like that set out in Table 2.1.

In this generalized formula, the function of the anionic detergent (1) is obvious, the function of the alkanolamide (7) is as a lather stabilizer, and the SCMC (3) is included to assist in the suspension of dirt particles, as was described in the section on laundry soaps.

Sodium tripolyphosphate (2), which forms a large proportion of

**Table 2.1**

|                                                      | *Percentage* |
| ---------------------------------------------------- | -----------: |
| 1. Sodium alkyl benzene sulfonate                    | 15.0 |
| 2. Sodium tripolyphosphate                           | 35.0 |
| 3. Sodium carboxymethyl cellulose (SCMC)             | 1.0 |
| 4. Sodium disilicate                                 | 2.5 |
| 5. Sodium perborate                                  | 25.0 |
| 6. Optical brightener                                | 0.1 |
| 7. Alkanolamide                                      | 1.5 |
| 8. Sodium sulfate to complete to . . . . . . . . . . . . . . . 100.0 per cent | |

modern detergent powders, is a close chemical relative of sodium hexa-metaphosphate, sold as a water softener under various trade names. It may seem strange at first to add a water softener to a formula using synthetic detergents, which are not much affected by hard water, but the action of the tripolyphosphate is much more complex than it first appears. It has been shown that, particularly in the cases of cotton and other cellulose fibers, solid dirt is held onto the fabric not only by grease, but by chemical bonds which include calcium and magnesium compounds. Water softening materials like sodium hexametaphosphate and sodium tripoly-phosphate act as softeners by removing calcium and magnesium com-pounds which could interfere with the performance of soap, and they can therefore also be used to remove the calcium and magnesium compounds which bind dirt to fabrics. They also assist in the removal of stains such as iron rust, blood, and so on, which involve metallic bonds between the colored material and the fiber.

Sodium hexametaphosphate would be quite suitable chemically for use in detergent powders, but in practice it tends to make the powders cake badly by picking up moisture from the air; sodium tripolyphosphate gives a very crisp free-flowing powder which does not absorb atmospheric moisture.

It has been considered in recent years that the phosphates in deter-gents might add to pollution hazards. This is not because they are harm-ful in themselves, but because they encourage the growth of water plants and algae in rivers and lakes, by simple fertilizer action. When such growth becomes so thick that the layer of algae stops aeration of the water, the state is known as *eutrophication*. After a conservationist campaign to stop the use of phosphates in detergents, some manufacturers removed them from their products. It now appears, according to later information, that the phosphates in detergents are unlikely to cause eutrophication, and they are regaining their place in washing products.

Sodium disilicate (4) is the silicate familiar in solution as "water-glass"; its use in detergent powders is the purely mechanical one of binding the powder ingredients into granules.

Sodium perborate (5) is a solid compound of hydrogen peroxide and sodium borate; it behaves as a source of hydrogen peroxide, but in a solid and stable form, and is therefore a bleaching agent. Hydrogen peroxide is safe with almost all fabrics, and is therefore the best bleach to use in general-purpose powders, but it has the great disadvantage that it is almost inactive at low temperatures, and needs a wash temperature of at least 60° C before it bleaches properly. This is satisfactory for washing machine use, but under conditions of hand washing in bowls and so on the sodium perborate added to detergent powders is entirely wasted. There is a great deal of research going on to produce a bleach that is as safe as sodium perborate but which acts at lower temperatures. Such an effect could be achieved either by inventing a new type of bleach or by activating the sodium perborate so as to make it effective at lower temperatures. Both lines of research are being pursued actively by the large detergent companies and other manufacturers.

The optical brightener (6) behaves in exactly the same manner as has already been described in the section on soap. It is found, however, that all optical brighteners act much more efficiently in synthetic detergent solutions than in soap solutions, and the brightening effect is consequently greater. Domestic powders usually contain a mixture of optical brighteners—those that are useful for cotton (c.s.f.a. = cotton-substantive fluorescent agents) are often far less efficient on synthetic fibers such as nylon, Orlon, and so on, and specially formulated optical brighteners have to be added to the powders to deal with these fibers. This is obviously an additional cost which may not be justified if the user is only going to wash cotton and other cellulosic fibers, and in some industrial versions of the detergent powders, the optical brighteners used are only c.s.f.a.'s, and not substantive on nylon and acrylic fibers.

Last, the sodium sulfate (8) is added for no other reason than that it is a neutral, harmless dry powder that will help to absorb the other ingredients of the powder.

The accepted method of manufacturing these powders is *spray drying*. All the ingredients except sodium perborate and perfume, which might be damaged by heat, are mixed together with water to form a slurry, and this is pumped through fine nozzles at the top of a tower. Hot air is swept up the tower so that each droplet of solution is dried on its way down, and dry powder can be taken away at the bottom of the tower. As each droplet tends to dry on the outside first, and then the interior moisture bursts out as steam, the granules produced are hollow, and therefore the bulk density of the powder is low. Sodium perborate and perfume are dosed into the powder as it is led away from the tower to the packing plant. Spray drying facilities for such a process are, as has been said, extremely expensive capital accumulations, and must be utilized as much as possible for profitable operation. The spray drying is itself quite a skilled operation, as quite minor changes in the composition of the slurry can cause the product to be sticky, or, on the other hand, too dry and crumbly. The ideal is a crisp uniform granule, and great precision in working is necessary to maintain this. For these reasons, formulas in this market change slowly, and a multiplicity of different products in the same tower is anathema to the production unit.

Powders can, of course, be made without spray drying, but there are two main objections to "dry-mixed" materials. It is difficult to stop the ingredients from separating again after they have been mixed, so that the heavier ingredients migrate to the bottom of the package, and they are usually denser than spray-dried material (because the granules are not hollow) so that users who are accustomed to estimate usage of powders by eye or volume will find the dry-mixed materials more wasteful than the spray-dried kind. An available compromise is to buy spray-dried sodium tripolyphosphate, spray-dried detergent (mixed with sodium sulfate), and so on, and mix these powders to make the required formula. This permits variations from the Procrustean needs of the household market, and many manufacturers are working along these lines.

Another type of detergent powder is the hard-surface cleanser, not designed for use on fabrics but only for surfaces such as paintwork, tiles, working surfaces, and so on. These products make use of the properties of sodium tripolyphosphate as a stain remover and "loosener" of solid dirt particles, and in this case the tripolyphosphate is the main cleanser, with only enough detergent added to give wetting action. The powders usually contain, in addition, alkali such as trisodium phosphate, which increases the efficiency of the product in removing grease. The main essential for such products is that the ingredients, if not properly rinsed away, should leave no visible residue; it is often impossible to rinse a hard surface properly. The claims that they *need* no rinsing are rather exaggerated, and on paintwork in particular the long-continued action of trisodium phosphate will tend to soften the paint. When such hard-surface cleansers are used, therefore, they should always be followed by wiping with a cloth or sponge dipped in clean water. They should not be used habitually on floorings which are sensitive to alkali, such as cork, linoleum, or magnesite, but the occasional use is justified because often, unfortunately, the only choice is between slight damage to the floor from a harsh cleanser or leaving it dirty!

Most of the specialized detergent powders made for machine dishwashing are of a type similar to hard-surface cleansers, but they are considered in detail in Chapter Ten, along with other aspects of dishwashing.

There are no universally recognized standards for detergent powders, although the A.S.T.M. gives methods of analysis. The buyer should remember that the cleansing action of the powders is due mainly to the detergent raw material, sodium alkyl benzene sulfonate, and the sodium tripolyphosphate, and other things being equal, a powder with more of either of these ingredients than the other will also be a better cleanser.

## DETERGENT LIQUIDS

For general cleaning and dishwashing, liquid detergents have become preferred, replacing soap powders and flakes almost entirely. Most of the liquids are based on sodium alkylbenzene sulfonates or similar anionic detergents, but these are blended with other materials to increase the lather of the detergents and also to increase their solubility in water.

Blends of alkylbenzene sulfonates and nonionic detergents are quite common, especially on the industrial market. Such a blend combines the best qualities of each type of detergent, and in fact it is found that mixtures in certain proportions show a better performance than would be expected from the average of the components. This effect is known as *synergism;* similar improved effects from combinations of materials are found in germicides, which are considered in the next chapter. The favored blend for liquid detergents is roughly two-thirds sodium alkyl benzene sulfonate, of the form suitable for liquid products, and one-third nonionic of the alkyl phenol polyoxyethylene type. Solutions can be made up to about 30 per cent active material; if higher concentrations are required it is necessary to use alcohol, urea, sodium toluene sulfonate, or similar solubilizing agents. These, of course, raise the cost of the liquid without adding to its detergency, but on the other hand a more concentrated detergent costs less to package per pound of active detergent material.

Nonionic detergents of the alkanolamide type may also be added to anionic detergents. These will increase the lathering power and the viscosity of the solution, thus making the product superficially more attractive. They do not add very much to the detergency.

Most of the domestic liquid detergents are made from a mixture of anionic detergents, usually alkyl benzene sulfonates as the main ingredient and alkyl ether sulfates or alkyl amide sulfates in sufficient proportions to give a high concentration of detergent (up to 45 per cent can be obtained by proper formulation), a high viscosity and a large amount of rich lather. Again, if very high concentrations of detergent are required, alcohol, area and other solubilizing agents can be added. Such formulas are probably quite suitable for normal dishwashing, which is really not a very exacting process, but their formulation tends to be such that most of the ingenuity of the manufacturers has gone into the superficial qualities of lather and viscosity. For an exacting job, blends of alkyl benzene sulfonate and polyethylene glycol type nonionics are to be preferred.

For many purposes, a very good result can be obtained with the polyethylene glycol type nonionics by themselves. They have the disadvantage, for the user, that the foam is always poor, so that it is difficult to tell when a bucket or sink full of detergent is exhausted, but they are excellent cleansers and grease removers, and for some purposes (e.g. in dishwashing and tray-washing machines) they may be far superior to foaming detergents, because too much foam can reduce the mechanical cleansing effect of the jets.

As a counterpart for the hard-surface cleansing powders, there are liquid detergents for similar purposes. These normally contain a small amount of anionic detergent as wetting agent and around 20 per cent sodium tripolyphosphate or the more soluble material, potassium pyrophosphate. They may also contain nonionic ingredients of the alkanolamide type, mainly to keep the other materials in solution or suspension. Some of these cleansers contain ammonia in small amounts. This is largely to give the *impression* of a powerful cleanser, as the amount of ammonia which can safely be included is very limited and would have no more effect than a very small amount of additional alkali of the conventional kind.

The difficulties of dissolving substantial quantities of tripolyphosphate in such products have led to the investigation of other materials with similar powers for removing calcium and magnesium compounds. Nitrilo-triacetic acid (NTA) and ethylene-diamine tetracetic acid (EDTA) are materials with this property that are very much more soluble in water than the polyphosphates. The choice of phosphates or NTA/EDTA is largely a matter of economics; there is no particular advantage in cleansing power possessed by one or the other group. The ecological problems are discussed in the previous section.

In general it should be noted that liquid detergents require only simple equipment for their manufacture, in contrast to the large and costly spray-drying towers required for powders. It is quite possible to make good liquid detergents with no more than a jacketed vessel and stirring equipment, and the small manufacturer can buy his raw materials (alkyl benzene sulfonates, etc.) from large suppliers and blend these to make detergents "tailored" for a particular customer or trade; many small manufacturers operate in this way. The buyer of liquid detergents can therefore have a good deal of choice, and can shop for the products exactly suited to his needs at competitive prices.

SCOURING POWDERS

Scourers combine abrasive and detergent to remove heavy soiling and suspend it in detergent solution long enough for it to be washed away easily. They nearly always also contain a bleaching agent, usually of the chlorine-producing type. This is not only for stain-removal; chlorine bleaches have the effect of attacking most types of organic material (fats, the tar from burned food, oxidized polishes, and similar deposits), and they consequently assist the abrasive in its primary task of removing the soiling from the surface. The ordinary scouring powder contains about 3 per cent of detergent, usually alkyl benzene sulfonate, about the same amount of sodium tripolyphosphate to assist in "lifting" the soil, enough chlorinating agent to give about 1-2 per cent of chlorine (this will probably be in the form of one of the chlorinated forms of isocyanuric acid. These materials are stable dry powders which contain large amounts of chlorine which they release when the powders are wetted or dissolved in water), and alkali such as sodium carbonate or sodium phosphate, and the remainder abrasive powder. At one time silica was favored as the abrasive for scouring powders, but it has now been realized that the manufacture of powders with silica can cause silicosis among the work-people in the manufacturer's premises, and feldspar or dolomite minerals are now used instead.

## SOLVENTS

For certain purposes solutions of detergents in water are inadequate for cleansing, and solvents have to be resorted to. This is a step to be taken with caution: solvents are all very much more expensive than water, or even any ordinary detergent solution; they may have solvent effects on materials such as plastics or paint that the user does *not* want to remove; and they may have fire or toxicity hazards.

There are many hundreds of different solvents, but in a work on general cleaning it would not be appropriate to list most of these because they are only of importance for specialized uses. The solvents important for ordinary cleaning practice are as follows.

### Alcohol

Alcohol, ethyl alcohol to the chemist, is readily available as industrial spirit. So that commercial alcohol shall not be diverted into the manufacture of duty-free liquor, it is mixed with various *denaturants,* usually including methyl alcohol ("wood spirit") which is very poisonous and very difficult to remove from the potable ethyl alcohol. For all cleaning purposes, such denatured spirit is meant when "alcohol" is specified.

Alcohol is a mobile liquid boiling at 172° F (78° C) and very volatile. It is highly flammable, and strict fire precautions must be observed when it is used for cleaning. Alcohol dissolves resins, shellac and similar compounds, waterproof inks, many dyestuffs, including those used in ballpoint pens and felt-tip pens, iodine, and the coloring matters of many plants, including currants and other fruit. It has no effect on starches or gums, such as occur in food spills, but it can be mixed with water or detergent solution in any proportions, and the mixture can then be used for mixed soilings. It is of little use for dissolving fats and oils (except castor oil), waxes, rubber, tar, or plastic adhesives, but it is correspondingly safe to use on rubber or plastic materials and surfaces without swelling or damaging them.

From the point of view of the operator, alcohol is reasonably safe, mild on the hands, although some people may find it drying to the skin, and not particularly poisonous. The vapor may cause intoxication in high concentrations, but there are no long-term effects, and with reasonable ventilation the solvent is safe to use.

### Acetone

This is a strong-smelling mobile liquid boiling at 133° F (56° C), very volatile and very flammable, so it should be treated with great respect. It dissolves resins, paint (including cellulose paints), cellulose acetate fabrics, lipstick, nail varnish, many dyestuffs and many plastic materials. Acetone can be mixed with water or detergent solutions; because of its effect on plastics and paint or varnish, it should be confined to inorganic surfaces such as concrete, magnesite or tiles. In any case, it should not be used except for emergency stain removal.

Acetone is fairly harmless to operators, except that it degreases the skin very thoroughly and may cause soreness. The vapor is rather overpowering and good ventilation is essential.

### Gasoline

This is the most volatile of the petroleum spirits usually encountered as a solvent. Gasoline will dissolve tar, rubber, wax, and pitch, but has little effect on paints or resins. In general it should be avoided because of the dangerous fire risk.

### White Spirit

This petroleum solvent is the fraction distilling between about 320° and 356° F (160° and 180° C), and, like gasoline, is a mixture of many different hydrocarbons. Its flammability is high, but not nearly as high as that of gasoline, and it dissolves similar materials—tar, rubber, fats, oils, wax, and pitch. It has very little effect on paint, resins, or plastics, but should never be used on a rubber surface because of its swelling effect on rubber.

White spirit is fairly harmless to the skin, except for a degreasing effect that may lead to soreness. Rubber gloves are obviously no use to protect the hands, and polythene gloves are little better, but a good "dry work" barrier cream will give some protection. The vapor may cause dizziness after long periods of work, but it is quite safe with adequate ventilation.

*Stoddard solvent* is a particular form of white spirit used by dry cleaners. It is slightly less volatile than the normal white spirit, and therefore a little less flammable.

### Kerosene

This is an even less volatile petroleum solvent. It is far less flammable than gasoline or white spirit, and will not ignite in bulk, only when spread out by a wick or on shavings, etc. It dissolves the same kinds of material as gasoline or white spirit, but more slowly.

None of the petroleum solvents is soluble in water or alcohol. They can be emulsified in certain specialized types of nonionic detergent solution, and this is the basis of many of the solvent/detergent blends that are made up for degreasing machine parts, etc., and for removing very heavy soiling with tar, oil, or rubber. In such products the solvent softens and dissolves the greasy material, and then the detergent carries away the mixture of grease and solvent as an emulsion, so that the last traces can be rinsed away with water.

### Carbon Tetrachloride

This is typical of the class of *chlorinated solvents,* in which some or all of the hydrogen atoms in a hydrocarbon material have been replaced by chlorine atoms. The effect is to increase the solvent power of the materials for grease and wax, etc., and at the same time to eliminate most of their flammability. Obviously this is only done at an increased cost, due to the expense of preparing the chlorine and incorporating it into the compounds.

Carbon tetrachloride is a heavy liquid (1 gallon weighs 13.2 pounds, compared with 8.3 pounds for a gallon of water or 6.6 pounds for white spirit) which is very volatile; it evaporates readily at room temperature and boils at 169° F (76.5° C). It is entirely non-flammable, and in fact smothers fires very effectively.

This solvent was once used very widely for dry cleaning and general cleaning, but it has been largely superseded because of two major safety objections: in the long-term use, the vapor can cause major liver damage, accompanied by loss of weight, nausea, and other unpleasant symptoms. This might not trouble those who are only required to use the solvent on rare occasions, but it is also dangerous because it can produce the toxic gas *phosgene* when heated. Inhalation of carbon tetrachloride vapor through a cigarette, for instance, can cause alarming lung damage from the effects of the phosgene.

### Trichlorethylene

This chlorinated solvent was developed in a search for less dangerous solvents than carbon tetrachloride. It is similar in appearance and smell, boils at 188° F (86.9° C), weighs about 12.2 pounds per gallon, and is non-flammable.

It dissolves all fats and waxes, oils, tar, pitch, paint, resin, rubber and many plastics. It should not be used on surfaces containing rubber, vinyl, pitchmastic, or bitumen, but confined to concrete, magnesite, and similar inorganic (mineral) surfaces. It can dissolve certain cellulose acetate fabrics and PVC, so care should be taken in dry-cleaning or spotting clothes.

Trichloroethylene is degreasing to the skin and usually makes it sore after prolonged contact; a good dry-work barrier cream will give some protection. The vapor is narcotic if breathed for very long, and can be dangerous in prolonged use. Ventilation should be good when this solvent is used.

### Tetrachloroethylene

This solvent is also called perchloroethylene. It is very similar to trichloroethylene, except that it boils at 250° F (121.2° C) and weighs 13.5 pounds per gallon. It is safer on synthetic fabrics than trichloroethylene and therefore preferred by dry cleaners.

### Methylene Chloride

This is the most volatile of the common chlorinated solvents; it boils at 41° C and thus tends to evaporate very quickly at room temperature. It weighs 11.1 pounds per gallon and is *flammable,* unlike the other chlorinated solvents.

Methylene chloride dissolves fats and waxes as do the other chlorinated solvents, but it is used in particular for its great speed in penetrating and softening paint films. Solvent paint strippers usually contain methylene chloride mixed with a synthetic gum, such as methylcellulose, to thicken the compound and slow down the evaporation of the solvent.

Methylene chloride is such a powerful solvent that it should never be used on, or even near, plastic, rubber, painted or varnished surfaces, unless it is intended that these should be stripped.

### Fluorinated Solvents

There is a large group of solvents similar to the chlorinated ones but having some of the chlorine atoms replaced by fluorine. These materials are very stable, non-toxic and volatile, and are used mainly for refrigerator fluids and propellents for aerosol cans. However, Freon 113 (E.I. du Pont de Nemours & Co),or trichlorotrifluoroethane, finds some use as a solvent. It behaves rather like trichloroethylene, but is milder in its action and safe on most plastics. It is non-poisonous and non-flammable. It is also, at present, very expensive.

## POLISHES

Polishes are products designed to give a smooth shiny finish to surfaces. They can achieve this in three ways:

1. Removing adherent dirt which is making the surface irregular.
2. Rubbing down minor imperfections in the surface itself, such as scratches or corrosion pitting.
3. Filling up minor imperfections and coating the surface with a layer of material that is itself smooth and shiny.

For instance, a glass polish, working on the hard, smooth surface of glass, is mainly the first type of polish, removing dirt and grease so that the clean surface of the glass can be seen. Brass, silver, and other metal polishes contain fine abrasive that rubs down the metal so as to cover up scratches and pits, so they are the second type of polish. A plastic or wax floor polish fills up the irregularities of the floor surface with a layer of plastic or wax material that is fluid enough to flow into a smooth layer. This is the third type of action. In practice, many polishes combine some or all of these functions, but the proportions to which they are cleansers, abrasives, or fillers may vary according to the product and the surface; polishes will therefore be classified according to the type of surface on which they are used.

### Floor Polishes

These are designed mainly for linoleum, cork, wood, PVC and other surfaces which can be roughened by wear and thus lose their gloss. The oldest type of formulation is the solid wax polish, or *wax paste*, which consists of a partial solution of wax in solvent; solid wax in excess of the solubility in the solvent forms a mass of solid crystals which hold the product in its pasty form.

For floors, the wax is really expected to do two jobs which are diametrically opposed. It must be easy to rub out into a smooth layer on the floor, but once there, it must resist pressure and sliding of feet and other traffic without marking or smearing. Obviously no one material can fulfill both these needs entirely satisfactorily. Very hard waxes of the carnauba and montan type give the best compromise.

Carnauba wax comes from the cera trees of South America, and about 40 million cera trees are needed to furnish the 11-12,000 tons of carnauba wax used annually (world-wide). Alternatives to carnauba are montan wax, curicuri wax, palm wax, sugar cane wax and other vegetable waxes, or beeswax, Chinese insect wax, and ghedda wax. They are all rather expensive, and the solution of beeswax in turpentine that was the standby of the nineteenth-century housewife is now hardly an economic proposition.

A polish made entirely from these hard waxes would not only be expensive but it would be very difficult to rub out to a smooth surface, even with the solvent to help by redissolving some of the wax during the rubbing process (waxes are more soluble in warm solvent than in cold, so the rubbing helps to dissolve the wax, which then reprecipitates on the surface as the solvent cools again). Softer waxes are added, such as paraffin wax, partly for economy and partly to make the wax easier to rub out onto the floor. They soften the final surface so that it marks more easily under pressure, but this in itself has some advantages, because the softer surface allows the feet to sink in very slightly, and the floor is for this reason less slippery than one coated with the hard glassy surface of carnauba wax alone. A more modern additive to wax pastes is polythene wax, a solvent-soluble form of the well-known plastic. This is extremely useful in reducing slip, as the polythene wax seems to take up a slightly granular form as it solidifies, making the surface more non-slip without too much loss of gloss.

Silicone oils added to wax pastes assist with the rubbing out process by liquefying the wax as it is rubbed, and lubricating its movement over the floor. Silicones do not help to make a hard surface, but their great repellency towards water helps to render the surface resistant to spills.

Wax pastes are still popular to some extent on the domestic market, but the labor involved in spreading the polish and then buffing it has virtually eliminated them from industrial practice in favor of the "dry bright" polishes. These are liquids that only need to be spread evenly over the floor, by mopping or spraying, and dry with the gloss already developed, with buffing. The simplest of such products is so-called "button polish," occasionally used as a sealing and polishing treatment for wood floors.

Button polish is a solution of shellac in alcohol, and is therefore very similar to a french polish formulation. The name has nothing to do with clothing, but arises from the fact that the shellac most suitable for making up the solution is produced in small round blobs or buttons, and is called "button lac."

Such a product, although cheap, is not entirely suitable for floor finishing. It tends to darken on exposure to light and air, it cannot be rebuffed if the surface is damaged, and the gloss is not very good. Industrial floor polishes and domestic "dry bright" polishes are therefore formulated from synthetic plastic materials which give a hard glossy surface when spread over the floor in the form of an emulsion in water. The two most widely used plastics are polystyrene and sodium or amine polyacrylates. If it is not necessary for the surface to be buffable—in fact, if any damage to the surface is to be repaired by reapplication of the plastic, then such an emulsion is all that is required, and many of the very inexpensive dry-bright polishes sold for contract work consist of nothing but polystyrene emulsion.

However, repeated applications of plastic, even if it is resistant to yellowing, tend to build up a layer of dirty polish which requires frequent stripping. For many purposes it is better to be able to run a polishing machine over the surface and restore the gloss by buffing. This requires the presence of some wax in the formulation. Resin may be added to help with the leveling, i.e. the initial spreading of the polish emulsion into a smooth layer. The uses of these various ingredients are summarized in Table 2.2.

### Table 2.2 The Ingredients of Floor Polishes

1. *Plastic materials*
   a) Polystyrene: high initial gloss, poor removability, low cost, powdering and yellowing on aging.
   b) Polyacrylates: fair initial gloss, good removability, very good resistance to yellowing and powdering. Resistant to water spotting. More expensive than polystyrene.
   c) Metallized polyacrylates: these contain zinc or zirconium compounds which link the molecules of plastic together, thus making a very tough and hard-wearing surface. Great resistance to yellowing, powdering, spotting, alkalis, solvents. Much more expensive than polystyrene—mainly used in specialty heavy-duty polishes.

**Table 2.2 (cont.)**

2. *Waxes*

   a) Hard waxes (carnauba, montan, etc.): high initial gloss, excellent durability, high cost, very slippery.
   b) Polythene waxes: fair initial gloss, moderate durability and buffability, some powdering, moderate cost.
   c) Soft waxes: poor initial gloss, moderate durability, easy buffability, good slip resistance, low cost.

3. *Resins*

   a) Ordinary resin: contributes to leveling, gloss and adhesion, alkali-soluble and therefore easily marked by soap, etc.
   b) Terpene resins: improve slip resistance, tend to be dark and to accelerate yellowing.

4. *Shellac*

   Added to improve adhesion to surface, levelling and gloss. Difficult to strip and tends to yellow.

5. *Colloidal silica*

   Added to improve slip resistance, removability and buffability. Tends to impair soil and scuff resistance.

6. *Plasticizers*

   These are high-boiling-point solvents, added to increase initial gloss and buffability. They impair scuff resistance and heel mark resistance.

7. *Silicones*

   These are derivatives of silica (sand, quartz) which has been chemically modified until it has lost its crystalline character and appears as oily liquids or waxes. These "silicones" still retain some of the characteristics of the silica parent, as they are very resistant to chemical attack, temperature, and other agencies. The consistency of a silicone oil will usually remain the same over a wide range or temperature, even -40° through 328° F (-40° C through 200° C). They are excellent lubricants, mainly because they have no chemical affinity with any type of surface and tend to "glide over" other materials. Added to polishes in small quantities (for cost and efficiency reasons), they enhance the water repellency and gloss of the surface. Usually mixture of a high-viscosity silicone and a low-viscosity one gives the best results.

8. *Fluorocarbons*

   These are materials of a fatty nature, containing fluorine instead of some or all of the hydrogen normally present in hydrocarbons. They behave in a way best described as "super waxes," being slippery, water-repellent, and oil repellent. The commonest of the group, poly-tetrafluoroethylene (PTFE) is well known as a lubricant and non-stick finish for saucepans and similar utensils. Fluorocarbons are used in small quantities because of their high cost.

With this choice of raw materials, the polish formulator makes up the best compromise for the purpose in hand within the price limitations set by the market. Obviously many of the ingredients are mutually antagonistic—shellac produces all the opposite characteristic to plasticizers, for instance—but by carefully balancing the properties of each ingredient, excellent products can be made.

In the industry, polishes of this type are usually classified into three types, depending on the balance of the ingredients. Polishes that dry bright to give a hard surface that cannot be modified by friction (for example, a pure shellac or polystyrene finish) are called *non-buffable.* Products which are based on plastic materials but contain enough wax to permit them to be rebuffed by machine (but not by hand, without excessive effort) are called *semibuffable,* and products where the shine can be restored by hand polishing are called *buffable.* The last must contain a large amount of wax, silicone, or plasticizer, or all of these.

Polishes made with metallized polyacrylates are resistant not only to water, but to ordinary alkali; they resist the action of most cleansing solutions. To remove this type of polish it is necessary to use either a special stripper containing ammonia, or to add an ounce or two of household ammonia to each gallon of detergent solution made up for cleaning.

For many purposes, the surface of a floor polished with semibuffable polish may be renewed by spraying the floor lightly with polish in dilute emulsion, and then buffing vigorously. This procedure may be carried out without previous washing if the floor is not too dirty, as the emulsion itself has some cleansing power. An extension of this idea, mainly for the domestic market, is the "cleaner-polish," which combines detergent and the ingredients of a dry-bright emulsion polish. The product is laid down on the floor using a damp mop, picking up the dirt in the process. The mop should be wrung out frequently during the polishing to remove the dirt. After the surface has been covered it is allowed to dry, as with the normal emulsion polishes.

The system is not very efficient. It has been estimated that, considering the two stages of cleaning and polishing, nine times as much of the solution is used in cleaning as is used in polishing, and therefore 90 per cent of the polish ingredients added to the product are literally poured down the drain with the dirty water. Secondly, the products do not in practice work well on a dirty floor, and the first polish coating is usually rather poor in gloss. Good results are only obtained with careful hand application in straight lines, which makes the products unsuitable for large areas where machine application is necessary. In general, therefore, it is better to use a two-stage approach, with an effective detergent to wash the floor followed by a good emulsion polish. The compromise product is more expensive and less efficient.

## Floor Sealers

One of the qualities which the polish formulator tries to achieve is good "hold-out"—the polish should not sink into the flooring excessively, otherwise it will be uneconomical. The user can also cut down the absorption of polish by making sure that the floor is suitably sealed with some cheaper material before polish is applied.

Seals for concrete and similar surfaces are usually made of rapidly drying oils, such as tung oil and other oleo-resinous materials. They behave like a quick-drying varnish. Superior results, with better abrasion resistance, are given by chlorinated rubber in suitable solvents, or polyacrylate or polyurethane preparations. These behave like a thin sheet of plastic over the concrete.

Wood, cork, linoleum, and similar absorbent surfaces should be sealed with tung oil, urea-formaldehyde resins, polyacrylates, or poly-urethanes, according to the weight of traffic they are required to carry. Details of the best methods of application are given in Chapter Six in separate sections for each type of flooring material.

## Furniture Polishes

These are nearly always versions of wax paste polishes—a solution of wax in white spirit or similar petroleum solvent, emulsified in water. As furniture is not expected to stand up to the same sort of wear as a floor, the waxes can be softer than the carnauba type, and more silicone oil can be added to make polishing easier. Many of these wax emulsions are now sold in aerosol cans, which makes it much easier to obtain an even layer of polish.

## Metal Polishes

Polishes for metals such as brass and silver usually contain a fine abrasive to rub down scratches and pits—whiting or diatomaceous earth is used, as a quite soft mineral is suitable. These are mixed with a small quantity of detergent to remove grease; ammonia, which removes the tarnish from silver very rapidly by chemical action; and often a water-soluble solvent of the ether type, all in a suitable solution in water. The wadding type of metal cleaner contains solvent, ammonia (or an amine) and a small amount of detergent absorbed on the surface of wadding, which itself acts as an abrasive.

Polishes for iron and steel objects (or, more normally, chromium-plated steel) need to remove rust marks from the surface of the metal. They usually contain phosphoric acid or an acid phosphate for this purpose, together with detergent, abrasive, and other materials.

# three

# Dermatitis and Cleaning Products

It is a very lucky management that has not, at some time, been faced by the problems of a case of dermatitis in a member of the staff, blamed on materials handled during the course of work. Because of the constant contact of cleaning materials with the hands, and the fact that these materials are not always used as carefully as they should be, such complaints are a hazard of the cleaning and maintenance business, whether for the office manager with a few cleaning personnel or the contract cleaner with hundreds. It may be useful, therefore, to outline the basic nature of dermatitis, the ways in which it may be caused, and the medical attitude to industrial dermatitis (insofar as *one* attitude exists).

Dermatitis means, quite simply, inflammation of the skin, and it can vary from a slight reddening, no worse than the effects of a rough shave, to acute swelling and eruption, accompanied by fever, which requires instant medical attention. The severe forms of dermatitis are spectacular in the degree of temporary disfigurement of the face, by swelling and cracking of the skin, and the complications may include severe skin infection from *Staphylococci* which enter the damaged skin, and various side effects from the raised temperature. Some people have died as the result of dermatitis, although the immediate cause of death is usually pneumonia, from the high temperature, or blood poisoning from secondary infections. In any case, it is obvious that dermatitis must be taken seriously.

There are three distinct causes of dermatitis which must be differentiated—primary irritation, photosensitization, and allergy.

## PRIMARY IRRITATION

This is due to simple damage of the skin cells, removal of essential materials from the skin, or otherwise gross interference with the working of the skin as a living organ. Caustic soda lye, for instance, dissolves skin cells away, leaving the sensitive underlayers exposed; petrol dissolves away the natural fat that protects and lubricates the cells; a layer of paint prevents the skin from losing moisture at the rate it requires to. All these effects have points in common; they always happen, in the sense that everybody reacts more or less (nobody is *allergic* to caustic soda because everyone is irritated by it; allergy is a personal peculiarity), they happen on the first occasion that the irritant is applied to the skin, and the degree of irritation is more or less proportional to the amount of the irritant which gets into contact with the skin.

Primary irritation is fairly easy to avoid. The materials which affect the skin in this way are well known, and the use of them is limited in cleaning products. Where it is necessary to use caustic, acid, or degreasing materials in a product, manufacturers give a warning on the package about the possible dangers, and rubber gloves, barrier creams, and so on can be issued to personnel. The borderline case is that of detergents themselves. Detergents are not irritant in the sense that they are caustic or dangerous chemicals, but when hands are wetted by detergent solutions, as with washers-up or laundry operatives, there is a danger that the skin may become dry and cracked—"dish-pan hands"—which seems to be due to interference by the detergent with the natural materials in the skin that keep the water-balance of the skin at the right level.

It is difficult to assess how widespread or serious this trouble really is. There are undoubtedly some people who are seriously affected by detergents, especially detergent powders, but these are probably a small percentage of the population. Detergent manufacturers find that the incidence of complaints about effects on the skin rises in the winter, probably because chapping and detergents do not go well together. In any case, while the effects of detergents may be distressing for cosmetic reasons, they are not serious irritations in the medical sense.

## PHOTOSENSITIZATION

There are some materials that, although they are not irritant to the skin on first contact, give rise to acute irritation if the skin is exposed to sunlight. It is as if they accelerated the normal process of sunburning by a large factor. The materials are mainly plant oils—oil of bergamot, oil of lime, wild parsley, milfoil, buttercup, mustard, figs and angelica are some of the agents known—but some sulfonamide drugs, acriflavin and eosin (used in lipsticks) have been shown to have similar effect. It is obviously rather difficult to trace irritation by such materials, as it may only appear irregularly—it is necessary for the material to be left on the skin *and* the skin exposed to sunlight. There may, therefore, be other materials which cause photosensitive effects which have not yet been discovered or detected.

Because the materials known to have this effect are mostly aromatic oils, it is likely that photosensitization from cleaning materials originates with the perfume. Perfumers take care to avoid the known sensitizers such as bergamot oil, but other materials may be used which react in this way.

## ALLERGY

Allergy is the most difficult form of dermatitis to avoid, because it arises from individual peculiarities of the people involved. The word allergy means, in fact, *altered* or *other* reaction, implying that the effects are not those to be expected from the majority of people. Apart from the individual reaction, the differences between an allergic dermatitis and a primary irritant dermatitis may be listed as follows:

1. Primary irritants cause inflammation only where they have been in contact with the skin, or for a short distance around. A sensitizer can cause inflammation on other parts of the body and may even spread to the whole skin surface from one small area of contact.
2. Primary irritants cause about the same amount of inflammation every time they touch the skin (assuming that the strength and amount of the irritant is the same). A sensitizer may cause no result the first time it comes into contact with the skin, then, on another occasion, considerable inflammation. Very often successive contacts cause worse results.
3. Allowing for a certain amount of human variation, everyone is irritated by primary irritants; some people may be able to tolerate, say, a 1 per cent solution of caustic soda for longer than others, but everyone is affected to some degree. With a sensitizer, most people are unaffected by quite a high concentration of the material, while the allergic person develops a serious dermatitis from very small amounts. Strawberries, seafood, and some other foodstuffs which are quite harmless to the bulk of the population will produce acute and even dangerous inflammation in sensitive subjects. The dyestuff para-phenylene-diamine can be handled without risk by most people (the writer has on occasion handled the solid material in bulk), yet there are people who are brought out in the most alarming skin eruptions by contact with a few drops of dilute solution of the dye.

The last point emphasizes the difficulty of avoiding dermatitis of allergic origin, because no one can say what is likely to be a sensitizer to some particular person. Cod liver oil, boracic acid, dextrin, olive oil, liquid paraffin and many other materials that are harmless or even beneficial to the skins of most people have been recorded as causing allergic dermatitis.

If a worker complains of dermatitis, and it is not immediately traceable either to a recognized skin disease or a primary irritant (encountered either at work or *during leisure*—remembering that lime, cement, soldering flux, washing soda, caustic lye, toilet cleansers, cleaning fluids, gasoline and other materials encountered in the home may be primary irritants), then a doctor should be asked to try to trace the cause of the irritation. This he will probably do by asking for small samples of all the materials which the patient has eaten or handled recently, both at work and in the home, with emphasis on anything new. If the symptoms are obviously those of *contact dermatitis* he may restrict himself to materials that have been handled. These he will apply in small quantities to the skin of the patient in a *patch test*. The sensitizer, if it has been found, will cause an acute reddening or swelling, whereas the other materials will probably have no effect. In such a test the patient's clothing should not be ignored, as a new material can come into contact with the skin in this way. Nearly every new textile fiber finds a handful of allergenic wearers, and a large number of cases (some years ago) of mysterious inflammations of women's thighs were traced eventually to the introduction of nickel plated parts on garter belts.

If the offending material is traced, it may be enough to make sure that the patient does not use it again. If there are several cases, or a particularly violent one, it may be necessary to consider the separate ingredients of the material and try to pinpoint the sensitizer. This, in the case of formulated products such as cleansers, requires co-operation with the manufacturers.

While allergic responses are often alarming in appearance, it is fortunate that they rarely give rise to any long-term effect (as long as precautions are taken against secondary infection). This is as well, from the legal point of view, because it is very difficult to fasten the blame for any particular allergic dermatitis on any individual or party. The responses are so individual that only one or two persons in a million may be affected, and the manufacturer would therefore have to test well over a million people even to find out the chances of allergy (as statisticians will know, the actual number of tests, to have even a reasonable chance of finding sensitive persons, would be far higher than this). The wholesaler or management who supply a product cannot be expected to detect a possible allergy where the manufacturer has failed to do so, and the user cannot be expected to know what is in the product he or she uses (except in the cases, not unknown, where persons have deliberately induced dermatitis with a substance or product which they know will affect them, in order to claim damages. This happened in several cases with the para-phenylene-diamine hair dyes, mentioned above).

Any list of "known allergens" would be found to include all those mentioned earlier, cod liver oil, olive oil, and so on, and a great many other everyday materials, so there is no future in trying to avoid known allergens altogether.

Essentially, allergy must be regarded as a small but unavoidable hazard of everyday life, both in work and leisure. If management is faced by a situation where a worker is allergic to any material handled in the job, it is good management to try to move the worker or eliminate the material. If they are faced by a claim that the dermatitis is their responsibility, they should engage a qualified dermatologist to investigate the claim, and remember that dermatitis can be caused at home as well as at work. They should certainly not be panicked into accepting that the cause is a detergent, or any other material, without expert confirmation.

# four

# Hygiene and Disinfection

Most people can see dirt (although there are some who seem willfully to close their eyes to it when they are responsible for causing it) and can assess fairly well whether a building or object is "clean." No such simple test exists to say whether a building is hygienic, using that word in its proper sense of "promoting health." Bacteria, molds, yeasts and viruses are all invisible to the naked eye, yet they can affect health either directly or by spoilage of food and drink. The maintenance manager must concern himself with these tiny creatures although he cannot see them.

The need for higher standards of hygiene is inseparable from modern society. We live in a crowded environment, and one, moreover, where people mix in a more complex way than in the past. Even under the very poor hygienic conditions of the last century, when infant mortality was very high, there was a strong chance that those who actually survived the first few years of life could then cope with most of the bacterial diseases they were likely to encounter—in the family group, or even the village, people developed an immunity to the "local" germs, and they were not exposed very often to strange organisms. Under modern urban conditions, the position is very different. The average worker will live with one group of people, his family; commute to and from work with another group; work with a third; lunch, perhaps, with a fourth group; and possibly relax in the evening with a fifth group. The process of mixing becomes more complex as urban life becomes more complex.

It is no coincidence that more cases of food poisoning result from institutional and restaurant meals than from meals prepared at home. The general standards of cleanliness in many homes would not be tolerated for an instant in the catering industry, but the members of a family become accustomed to their "own" germs, and are not nearly as badly affected by unhygienic practices as they would be outside the home. This is a serious problem in the catering industry, as workers are likely to think that the hygiene rules imposed by the management are exaggerated and fussy—they reason that, because they and their family have never suffered any ill effects from, say, sneezing over food, it can do no harm. They forget, or just do not know, that germs that are harmless in the nose can cause illness or even death to someone not accustomed to this particular germ.

It is almost impossible to assess the real cost of infections, and equally impossible to say which of them are avoidable, but it is quite certain that many of them *are* avoidable, and the cost is far too high. The record of "incidents" of food poisoning is only the tip of the iceberg—outbreaks that are serious enough to attract the attention of the public health officers—and does not include all the cases of vague "stomach trouble" which pass unrecorded. Add to cases of food poisoning the enormous number of other infections—minor accidents that become complicated by suppuration, skin eruptions, athlete's foot and other fungus diseases, and so on. We cannot hope as yet to eradicate coughs and colds, but many of the complications which lead to loss of working time are due to secondary infections that could have been avoided if the sufferers had worked and lived in a more hygienic environment. The economic effects of a single outbreak of food poisoning can be enormous: the episode of a bakery in 1966 is an object lesson. The workers went out for their annual celebration in a bus party and had a meal together. Unfortunately, one of the staff serving the meal harbored the food poisoning organism *Salmonella anatum,* without herself suffering any ill effects; she was presumably immune to an organism she had harbored for years. The bakery workers became infected, and carried the organism home to their own factory. Very soon, food poisoning outbreaks occurred in the district, and these were traced to the bakery products. In consequence, the bakery had to be closed for three months while the workers gradually eliminated the germs—a catastrophic loss to the bakery owners. Hygiene is not a refinement or luxury in any industry—it is part of good management.

Not all dangerous germs are health hazards. Bacteria and molds can cause spoilage of food products, toiletries, textiles (mildew is a kind of mold), books and other print, paint, timber and leather. Effluent and sewage systems can become blocked by growths of bacteria and molds. A few years ago, for example, a plating plant with its own effluent system found that the equipment was completely blocked by a type of mold that was growing luxuriantly on solutions of the (normally) deadly poison potassium cyanide. None of these expensive losses, in health or industrial efficiency, can be avoided by cleaning alone—there must be positive action against the causative germs.

Bacteriology, in which we may include mycology, the study of molds or fungi, and virology, the study of viruses, is such a huge subject that no attempt can be made here to give any extended account. However, a few notes may help to explain the problems faced by the bacteriologist in following the behavior of germs generally ("germs" is an excellent vague word which can cover bacteria, molds, yeasts, and all other micro-organisms) and explain the methods used to control them.

There are many thousands of types of bacteria, molds, and so on, and most of them have to be described as the naturalist describes birds and animals, in terms of a species name and varieties within that species. This gives rise to some rather daunting names for quite common bacteria, and these names are sometimes used by the product suppliers, one suspects, rather to impress than to explain. A few simple definitions may clarify the situation.

## Bacteria

These are microscopic plants, with one cell. They vary very much in size, but on the average they are about one thousandth of a millimeter across, so that a period in this book could cover about a quarter of a million of them. Bacteria are classified into four main types according to their appearance when seen in the microscope. *Cocci* are round, *bacilli* are rod- or sausage-shaped, *spirilla* are spiral or S-shaped, and *vibrios* are comma-shaped. Within these classes the various members are named by their appearance, their habits (for instance, *Bacillus anthracis* is a rod-shaped organism that causes anthrax), or their method of grouping (*Streptococci* are round bacteria that hang together in bent chains—Greek *streptos,* flexible—while *Staphylococci* are round bacteria that hang together in bunches—Greek *staphyle,* a bunch of grapes. *Staphylococcus aureus,* which causes many skin eruptions such as boils, occurs as round *yellow* bacteria in bunches, and so on). The names are clumsy, but the principle is the same as that of the naturalist who calls a species, say, the red-headed woodpecker, thus defining it by its appearance and its behavior.

Given the moisture they need (in soil at least 5 per cent and preferably above 25 per cent) and a supply of food, bacteria can multiply inconceivably quickly. At a favorable temperature, one bacterial cell can split into two in as little as 20 minutes, these two into four in another 20 minutes, and four into eight by the time an hour has passed from the original single cell. If this multiplication went on at a constant rate, one cell could produce $2^{72}$ or about 5,000,000,000,000,000,000,000 offspring per day. Fortunately for every other living thing on earth, the ideal conditions are never achieved, mainly because the food supply for such an enormous number of bacteria could not possibly be accessible to them all if they were in one huge colony. However, it underlines the speed with which bacteria can multiply even under non-ideal conditions, and the way in which an apparently insignificant degree of contamination can lead to widespread infection if the conditions are just right for the bacteria and wrong for the human beings.

Most bacteria, of course, are quite harmless, and indeed beneficial to man. Most of the types, and by far the greatest numbers, are found in the soil, breaking down discarded vegetable matter, absorbing nitrogen, and doing other things that help to increase the fertility of the soil. Others are of importance only in food processing: the bacillus *Acetobacter aceti,* for instance, which turns alcohol to acetic acid, is a nuisance to brewers and wine makers, but a friend to the vinegar manufacturer. Relatively few are in fact dangerous to man, but unfortunately the only course open to the maintenance manager, faced by an invisible collection of bacteria, some of which are harmless and others dangerous, is to try to destroy all of them.

The various types are also differentiated by their methods of resisting attack. Some are relatively easily killed by heat or sanitizers; others produce *spores,* which are a kind of quiescent form of the bacterium in a thick casing, with great resistance to attack. The spore cannot multiply itself, but it can survive a surprising amount of heat, cold, or chemical attack, and then, when conditions are favorable again, it sheds its "coat" and returns to its normal form (and starts multiplying again). The bacteriologist also divides bacteria into groups according to their response to staining with dyestuffs (a necessary stage in making them visible for microscopical work) and refers to "Gram positive" and "Gram negative" bacteria, according to their reaction to the stain invented by the bacteriologist Gram. The distinction is of no great importance to non-bacteriologists, but the phrases are often used in technical literature about sanitizing products.

## Molds

These are usually associated with growths on bread and other foodstuffs, and molds are in fact a very serious source of food spoilage. There are also molds that attack human beings directly, for example *Trichophyton purpureum* and *Trichophyton gypseum,* that cause athlete's foot, and the various *Microspora* that cause ringworm on the scalp. Molds do not multiply by the same simple cell division method as bacteria, and do not normally reproduce as fast, but on the other hand they need less moisture to survive, and in general the individual mold organism tends to have great powers of survival. The National Aeronautics and Space

Administration reported in 1967 that molds had been detected in the atmosphere at an altitude of 135,000 feet, apparently surviving the intense cold and virtual lack of any nourishment. Molds are classified in the same way as bacteria, except that the number of characteristic shapes is much greater.

## Yeasts

Yeasts are very similar to molds and other fungi, but the name is usually reserved for those organisms that ferment sugars. They are not harmful to human beings as a rule, although they may account for some skin inflammations and infections of the mouth and urinary system, but in brewing, wine-making and the food trade generally, the presence of airborne or "wild" yeasts can cause spoilage of materials containing sugar.

## Viruses

These contain the same type of material as the inside of the bacterial cell, but they have no cell-wall proper. They are considered on the borderline between the "living" bacterium and the "non-living" protein, in that they can multiply, or at any rate become multiplied, by putting together simpler substances and producing a duplicate of their own structure. On the other hand, they appear to have no viable existence if they are removed from close proximity with "living" organisms such as bacteria, plants, or animals. Viruses, being smaller and simpler than bacteria, can penetrate where bacteria cannot. They were first discovered because they penetrated filters used by early bacteriologists to strain off bacteria from their products, and this ability to enter the organs of animals with such ease may explain why some virus diseases, such as influenza, are so difficult to eradicate from the system.

## PATHOGENIC ORGANISMS

From the point of view of the maintenance manager, medical officer and all others interested in hygiene, the most important of all the foregoing organisms are those that produce diseases, the pathogenic organisms. The most important of these (in that the diseases are more or less serious and the bacteria are widespread) are as follows:

Various *Staphylococci. Staphylococcus aureus* is a common source of skin troubles such as abscesses, boils, and suppurating wounds. Internally it can cause peritonitis and other serious inflammations. *Staphlyococcus aureus* needs to penetrate the skin to lead to these troubles, but any small wound or sore place is sufficient to allow the germs to enter. Most people have quantities of *Staphylococci* in their noses and throats, and infection from this source arises very easily.

*Streptococci.* These are also sources of illness, very often the serious inflammations of internal organs. *Streptococcus viridans* is a cause of intestinal disorders and sore throats, and is very widespread.

*Salmonella typhimurium.* This organism is one of the most frequent and serious causes of food poisoning; the effects can easily be fatal if the bacteria have grown in food to any extent. Meat products, especially pork preparations, are likely to harbor *Salmonellae,* and they can only be killed by strict attention to hygiene and adequate cooking.

*Bacillus tuberculosis* or *Mycobacterium tuberculosis,* as its name suggests, is the cause of pulmonary tuberculosis. It is carried in sputum and has great powers of survival against unfavorable conditions and even many germicides. Fortunately the rise in standards of public hygiene and determined efforts to detect and treat tuberculosis in the early stages (X-rays and so on) have cut down the numbers of this organism in advanced countries, compared with the situation some years ago.

*Bacillus subtilis* is a common organism which is usually harmless. If it penetrates wounds it can exercise its proteolytic action in the bloodstream and cause poisoning.

*Pseudomonas* organisms are again common and usually harmless— they occur in enormous numbers in water and the soil. If they penetrate a wound the infection may be very hard to eradicate. *Pseudomonas pyocyanea* and *Pseudomonas aeruginosa* cause serious trouble in dirty wounds, such as those incurred in the building trade and on the battlefield; "gas gangrene" is a *Pseudomonas* infection of this kind.

*Escherichia coli* is an organism found in enormous numbers in the human bowel, particularly the colon, hence the name; it is not particularly dangerous, although it can give rise to inflammation if it penetrates to other body cavities (cystitis is usually caused by *Escherichia coli*). However, as it comes from the bowel, bacteriologists carrying out tests to assess the hygienic standards of premises or equipment look for *Escherichia coli* and other bowel bacteria, as the presence of these is good evidence of contamination from sewage, workers with poor standards of hygiene, and similar sources of trouble.

The bacteriologist carrying out quantitative work has problems which make his science far less exact than, say, chemistry or physics. First, it is very difficult to count the actual numbers of bacteria on a surface (for example, before and after treatment with a sanitizer), and what the bacteriologist actually does is to swab the surface in a controlled way, so as to pick up a fair sample of all the bacteria present, and then allow these to grow on a suitable source of food until they have multiplied into colonies that can be seen. This process is obviously open to serious errors in the swabbing, the "plating-out" onto a suitable food supply, the accuracy of the counting, and the chance that the bacteria may not always multiply in exactly the same way every time.

Secondly, it is not always feasible, or safe, to carry out tests with the really dangerous pathogenic organisms; unless the bacteriologist is actually working on treatements for cholera, for example, he is not likely to expose himself and his colleagues to the danger of working with the cholera vibrio, and any conclusions he draws about the effectiveness of a sanitizer or similar product are only valid for the organisms actually used in the tests.

Because of this type of approximation, the sensible bacteriologist does not pretend to a greater degree of exactness that he can really achieve; often results are expressed as simple approximations such as + (effective) or - (not effective), with ++ and +++ for greater percentage kills. Alternatively, results may be expressed as a 99 per cent kill or a 99.99 per cent kill, the latter usually meaning that the bacteriologist did not find any living bacteria, but allowing for the few that could have been missed. Bacteriological tests that are expressed with a high degree of accuracy, such as "57.4 per cent kill," should be treated as suspect. It is virtually certain that a test giving 57.4 per cent, if repeated, could give any result from 50 to 60 per cent.

## GERMICIDAL PRODUCTS

With the foregoing reservations, it is possible to describe the advantages and disadvantages of the many germicidal materials available to assist the maintenance manager in controlling the hygiene of his premises. There are many terms used in describing these, and the following glossary may be useful:

| | |
|---|---|
| **germicide** | Any material that kills bacteria, molds, or yeasts. It is a convenient general word. |
| **bactericide** | A material that kills bacteria, but not necessarily other organisms. |
| **bacteriostat** | A material that does not necessarily kill bacteria, but provides such an unfavorable environment that they do not multiply, or alternatively it kills them at about the same rate as they multiply. |

| | |
|---|---|
| **fungicide** | A material that kills molds, but not necessarily bacteria. |
| **fungistat** | A material that prevents molds from multiplying. |
| **antibiotic** | A material that kills bacteria by interfering with their metabolism, usually only in the body. |
| **antiseptic** | A germicide for use specifically on the body. |
| **sanitizer** | A germicide for use on surfaces, equipment, etc., and not usually on the body. |
| **preservative** | A material added to other products to kill germs that cause spoilage, not necessarily to protect the user against pathogenic germs. |

Many substances will, of course, fall into two or more of these classifications, according to circumstances. Some bactericides are also fungicides; some bactericides at very low concentrations are only bacteriostats; some sanitizers are safe enough on the skin to be antiseptics, and so on.

## TYPES OF GERMICIDE

### Phenols

Phenols are one of the oldest types of germicide used deliberately for hygiene purposes. When Lister commenced antiseptic surgery in 1865 he used phenol, or carbolic acid, as the bactericide, and it has retained a place in germ killing ever since. Phenol at 0.2-1.0 per cent is bacteriostatic for most organisms, while above 1.0 per cent it is bactericidal. Organisms that produce spores can usually survive the effects of phenol (*Bacillus anthracis*, that occurs in hides and hair and causes anthrax, has been known to survive for 24 hours in 5 per cent phenol).

*Cresol* is similar to phenol, having a slightly more tarry smell, reminiscent of the coal-tar from which both are derived. Neither phenol nor cresol is very soluble in water, but they can be dispersed in soap solution, and a solution of 50 per cent cresol in linseed oil soap solution is known as Lysol.

The main disadvantages of these materials are:

1. The strong tarry odor.
2. The high concentrations needed for a true bactericidal effect.
3. The corrosive effect of solutions of phenols on the skin and stomach, so that really effective phenol germicides tend to be irritant and poisonous.

They are, however, still used for such purposes as treating drains and sinks. "Black fluids" are emulsions of crude cresol in soap, and are black, oily, and strong-smelling; "white fluids" are lysol-like emulsions of refined phenols.

Slightly more complex phenols have similar bactericidal effects without such corrosive effects on the skin or mucous membrane. *Amyl cresol* is used mainly as a mouthwash and for similar antiseptic purposes, and *ortho-phenyl phenol* is used as a preservative for creams and similar products.

## Chlorinated Phenols

It was discovered in the last century that treatment of phenols to incorporate chlorine in the molecule increased the bactericidal action without increasing the poisonous or corrosive effects; in consequence, the new materials could be used at far lower concentrations and still be effective and safe. Such chlorinated phenols are now used extensively.

*Parachlorometa-cresol* (PCMC) is typical of the class. It is a crystalline powder, not very soluble in water, but dispersible in soap solutions. It has a strong phenolic odor, sharper than that of phenol or cresol. It is active against *Streptococci* in particular, less so against *Staphylococci*, and almost inactive against *Pseudomonas aeruginosa* and *Proteus vulgaris*, two common water- and soil-borne organisms. On the other hand, for general use, it has quite good fungicidal effects, and kills molds and yeasts, and also algae in water, which may be useful where water has to be taken from ponds or wells. PCMC is about 25 times as effective as an equal weight of phenol, when used in soap solution. This figure is given by the test invented by Rideal and Walker, now a standard test for all types of bactericide. The Rideal-Walker test compares bactericides against pure phenol in their action on the pathogenic organism *Bacterium typhosum* in a controlled way. The test is widely quoted to compare various proprietary products, and is certainly a reasonable approximation to an analytical standard. However, it must be remembered that the Rideal-Walker test is only carried out on one organism, and products which are extremely effective against *Bactenum typhosum* may be less effective against other organisms, and vice versa. Many manufacturers quote the results in the simplified terms "R.-W. 4-5" and so on. The range of figures represents the kind of reasonable caution that, as has been said, should be exercised when quoting bacteriological results.

*Parachloro-meta-xylenol* (PCMX) or just chloroxylenol, is similar to PCMC. It is used widely in antiseptics (in a similar soap solution—its solubility in water is even lower that that of PCMC).

*Dichloro-meta-xylenol* (DCMX) is an even more effective bactericide than PCMC or PCMX, and has some action against *Pseudomonas* organisms. It is even less soluble in water than PCMX, less than 1 part in 5000 at room temperature, but it can be dispersed in soap solution.

All these chlorinated phenols, when sold as antiseptics, are dispersed in soap. When the solution is diluted with water, the soap solution is no longer able to dissolve as much of the phenol, and this comes out of solution as a cloud of tiny droplets. This explains the well-known characteristic of these antiseptics of giving a cloudy white solution when diluted.

### Complex Phenols

Related to the simple chlorinated phenols, but more chemically complex, is a group of germicides that has considerable importance in the soap and cleansing industries, and also in toiletries. These were developed for use in toilet soap, but have since been used in many other types of products.

*Vancide BN* (a commercial trade name) is actually disodium 2,2'-thiobis (4,6-dichlorophenoxide). It is successfully used not only in toilet soap but in general cleaners, where its ability to remain on a surface after rinsing gives a much longer contact time and greater effectiveness against bacteria than with the simpler chlorinated phenols. Vancide BN is substantive to many textiles, and can be added to rug detergents, laundry products, and similar formulations at about 0.25 per cent to give a useful degree of sanitization.

Vancide BN has a tendency to darken in products when exposed to sunlight, and although this is not a serious disadvantage in itself, it tends to spoil the appearance of the products and may lead the purchaser to suppose that serious spoilage has taken place. A product of the complex phenol type which is free from this trouble, and therefore of interest to manufacturers of cleansing products, is *trichlorocarbanilide,* or TCC (properly 3,4,4'-trichlorocarbanilide), which shows no tendency to discolor in the light. It has been used widely in toiletries with antiseptic action, and is finding its way into the formulation of general cleaning products.

### CATIONIC GERMICIDES

In the last chapter, it was explained that cationic detergents possessed the same general characteristics as soap or other synthetic detergents: they reduce the surface tension of water so that it wets surfaces more effectively and can thus penetrate under greasy soiling, they foam, and they have some powers of suspending dirt particles and emulsifying grease. However, they do not, as a class, do any of these things very well, and as detergents alone they would have little or no importance except as laboratory curiosities. Cationics redeem themselves for practical purposes by possessing one important property that is not shared by other types of detergent to any extent—they kill bacteria.

The action of cationic detergents on bacteria is not very well understood. Phenols, and many other germicides, possess their germ-killing properties by virtue of poisoning the organisms. Bacteria absorb all their nourishment through their cell walls, having no "mouths," and they absorb phenols and similar material with their other food. Once inside the bacterial cell, the germicide stops one or other of the vital chemical processes that keep the organisms alive. Antibiotics, in general, also act in this way, and their chemical structures are carefully and ingeniously designed to make sure that they *are* absorbed. Cationic detergents, on the other hand, do not appear to penetrate the cell wall at all, but remain attached to the outside of it. Presumably they interfere with the taking in of food through the cell wall, a kind of siege warfare.

The point is not just of importance to bacteriologists. There are certain peculiarities in the action of cationic detergents on bacteria which can only be understood fully if it is appreciated that their mode of action is unusual, and not the same as that of most types of germicide. These points will emerge in discussion of the most important members of the cationic class.

*Cetrimide* (Myristyl trimethyl ammonium bromide mixed with small amounts of the similar materials cetyl trimethyl ammonium bromide and the stearyl compound) is a white crystalline powder, reasonably soluble in water to give a foaming solution. This is one of the oldest-established and most widely used of the cationic germicides, and is a quaternary ammonium compound—the myristyl group is the fatty part of the molecule, and the ammonia derivative the water-soluble group, hence the detergency of the material.

Cetrimide is very effective against *Staphylococci* and *Streptococci,* not so effective against some other types of bacteria, notably *Pseudomonas aeruginosa* and *Mycobacterium tuberculosis,* which seems to be able to survive quite large doses of concentrated Cetrimide solution. It is ineffective against spores. In sharp contrast with the phenolic type of germicide, it is almost odorless, colorless, and very mild in its action on the skin (Cetrimide is used widely for making up solutions for use on the skins of babies, for diaper rash, etc.) and it is therefore very much acceptable both for personal use and for use in food preparation areas, where the strong smell of PCMX, for example, would be quite out of place. Cetrimide is also effective at very low concentrations: 1 part in 5000 makes quite an efficient germicidal solution.

Because of the curious mode of action of cationic germicides mentioned above, it is found that *very* low concentrations of cetrimide, and other cationics, are bacteriostatic. It appears that even a trace of cetrimide in water will interfere with the cell walls of bacteria enough to make them go into a quiescent state and cease multiplying. When the germicide is washed away, however, the bacteria revert to their normal behavior. This peculiarity has led to some very variable results with cationics generally, some workers praising them for the apparent destruction of bacteria at incredibly low dosages, others condemning them because they have found bacteria still alive after several hours of exposure to the germicides. This is natural; bacteriologists, as has been said, assess the numbers of bacteria by letting them multiply and counting the colonies produced. If the germs are not in a mood to multiply, they are normally considered "dead," but of course they may revert to their normal habits if the circumstances change. The lesson to be learned is that cationics must be used at adequate concentrations, and too low a dosage may lead to situations where a surface is still contaminated although superficial tests show no active bacteria.

Cetrimide and other cationic germicides are attracted to all surfaces, not just those of bacteria or objects that are to be cleaned. If the germicides are used in circumstances where there is a large excess of solid material—debris, clay, textile fibers, etc.—allowance must be made for the amount of cationic that will be taken up by these materials. On the other hand, this attachment to surfaces can be used to great advantage in retaining some germicide on a surface after washing; thus, if blankets are rinsed in a solution of cetrimide, they will take up a coating of germicide that persists after further rinsing with water.

Cationics are also rendered inactive by several materials that react with them: soaps and anionic detergents are quite incompatible with cationics, and inactivate them almost entirely. So do phenols (so cationic germicides should not be mixed with phenolic germicides). Polyphosphate water-softeners and proteins also interfere (serum affects the action of cetrimide when it is used for dressing wounds). Nonionic detergents do not interfere as much as soap or anionic detergents, but it has been shown that they have some diminishing effect on the germicidal powers of cationics, and this again must be allowed for in the dosages recommended or used with mixtures of nonionics and cationics, which are widely sold as germicidal detergents.

*Benzalkonium chloride* (a mixture of various alkyl dimethyl benzyl ammonium chlorides) is another widely-used cationic germicide. It is usually supplied as a 50 per cent solution in water with a sirupy consistency and a peculiar smell, slightly reminiscent of bitter almonds. It is a more powerful germicide than cetrimide and has greater effectiveness against *Escherichia coli* and similar organisms—about 1½ times the effectiveness, according to one set of tests. One part of the 50 per cent material in 3000 parts of water makes an excellent germicidal solution.

The same limitations apply to bensalkonium chloride as to cetrimide; if anything, it is more sensitive to interference by soap and anionic detergents. It is active against *Pseudomonas aeruginosa* at 1 part in 5000 of 100 per cent material (i.e. 1 part in 2500 of the normal 50 per cent commercial product) given about one hour contact time, but at 1 in 10,000 at least nine hours' contact would be needed. Like cetrimide, it is relatively ineffective against fungi; the author has seen quite healthy colonies of mold *growing* in a 1 per cent solution of benzalkonium chloride which had been left standing for several weeks.

For the manufacture of cleansing products, benzalkonium chloride has two major advantages over cetrimide: it is cheaper in terms of effective concentrations, and it is very soluble in water, and therefore easy to blend. Many manufacturers now supply the raw material to Pharmacopoeia standard, so it would be invidious to pick out brand names.

*Cetyl pyridinium chloride* is a similar material to cetrimide. Although not strictly a quaternary ammonium compound, it is conveniently classified with them. Its properties are very similar to those of cetrimide, both in bacteriological effectiveness and solubility, etc. It is often used in medicine.

*Domiphen bromide* (lauryl dimethyl phenoxyethyl ammonium bromide) is a similar material to benzalkonium chloride—very soluble in water, rather more active than cetrimide against some of the *Pseudomonas* organisms, and effective at low concentrations.

*Hyamine 2389* (Rohm and Haas Corp.) or mixed alkyl tolyl trimethyl ammonium chlorides, is again similar to benzalkonium chloride. Table 4.1 indicates the level at which the product is (1) bacteriostatic, and (2) bactericidal.

With some organisms the difference in level is striking, showing again the partial effectiveness of cationics at very low concentrations.

Table 4.1

| Organism | Lowest concentration bacteriostatic | Lowest concentration bactericidal |
|---|---|---|
| Staphyococcus pyogenes | 1:4,000,000 | 1:1,000,000 |
| Staphylococcus aureus | 1:1,000,000 | 1: 512,000 |
| Bacillus suis | 1: 256,000 | 1: 128,000 |
| Salmonella typhosa | 1: 32,000 | 1: 32,000 |
| Proteus vulgaris | 1: 4,000 | 1: 2,000 |
| Pseudomonas aeruginosa | 1: 8,000 | 1: 2,000 |

Of course, these results were obtained under ideal conditions, and such very low concentrations would immediately fall off in efficiency in the presence of traces of any interfering substances, and the practical levels of germicide need to be several times larger.

*Dequalinium acetate* or strictly decamethylene-di-(4-amino-quinaldinium acetate) is related to the quaternary ammonium compounds, though not strictly chemically of this class. It represents one of a group of cationics which have been developed to deal with the main weakness of the common cationic germicides, their lack of effectiveness against molds and fungi. Dequalinium acetate is extremely potent against *Staphylococci* and *Streptococci,* and has some effect on *Pseudomonas* and similar organisms, but it is also effective against such fungi as *Candida albicans, Treponema vincenti* and other skin fungi such as the *Trichophyton* group that causes athlete's foot. The material is rather expensive, and so far is not used in general cleaning products, but it has great utility in lotions, creams, and other personal products for treating fungous diseases. A suitably priced cleanser containing this material or a similar fungicide would be very desirable for swimming pools, shower rooms, washrooms, and other places where athlete's foot fungi, in particular, tend to proliferate. Another salt of the same cationic, dequalinium chloride, is also available, but it is far less soluble in water than the acetate, and therefore more difficult to incorporate in products. It has the same effects, however.

*Chlorhexidine digluconate* (or 16-parachlorphenyl-diguanido-hexane-digluconate) is another compound related to the quaternary ammonium salts, but not quite the same chemically. It has striking activity against a wide range of bacteria, including many of the organisms not affected by normal cationics, and is finding increasing use in hygiene products for general cleaning. The material was first introduced as the chloride, but the solubility of this salt was too low for normal purposes and the gluconate, which is soluble in water up to 20 per cent, is now used more widely.

*Dioctyl- and didecyl-dimethyl ammonium bromides* are cationics which contain, instead of one fatty chain, two short ones. They are powerful germicides, and less affected by interference from anionic detergents, etc., than the compounds with one longer fatty chain, and are therefore better suited for general cleaning. They are used widely in breweries, canneries, and dairies, and are now being introduced widely into cleaning compositions.

Compounds with two *long* fatty chains in a quaternary ammonium compound are not very soluble in water, but find widespread use as softening agents and conditioners for fabrics. Distearyl dimethyl ammonium chloride, for instance, gives a very soft handle to wool. These materials have rather poor germicidal action.

CHLORINATING AGENTS

Chlorine is a heavy, greenish gas, very poisonous, with powerful bleaching and oxidizing effects. It reacts violently with some materials, and tends to attack all organic matter (i.e. those that are derived from living organisms or synthetic materials of a related type). It bleaches cotton, for instance, by virtue of the fact that it attacks the coloring matters (whether natural or dyestuffs) more rapidly than it attacks the cotton; however, it will attack the cotton also, given enough time. Woolen materials cannot be bleached with chlorine because in this case the fabric tends to be attacked faster than the coloring matter. It attacks the skin, the lungs (hence its use as a poison gas in World War I), and it also attacks bacteria, molds, yeasts, and viruses. Chlorine is thus a very powerful germicide, but not at all a specific one, because its mode of action is gross damage to the organism. If phenols and similar germicides act as poisons and cationic germicides by a kind of suffocation, one could say that chlorine kills by beheading and quartering.

Where it can safely be used, and this is the major limitation, chlorine is thus the most useful germicide which can deal with all kinds of micro-organisms. It has the widest range of killing power, against almost all living material, of any of the germicidal agents we shall consider in this chapter.

Chlorine does not normally act as a bleach or germicide in the absence of water, although the dry gas is still very reactive. In most cases, enough water is present for the chlorine to react with the water first, giving oxygen in a very active state, and chlorides, which are inactive. It is therefore the active oxygen which in fact bleaches and disinfects.

Chlorine gas is used in enormous quantities for public health purposes, mainly the treatment of water for domestic supply and in swimming pools. The treatment of these large volumes of water justifies the expense of the equipment for dosing chlorine gas accurately and safely; this would be too expensive and difficult on the small scale, so more convenient sources of chlorine have been evolved.

*Bleaching powder* (chloride of lime) properly called calcium hypo-chlorite, was the first of such materials developed, mainly for the bleaching of textiles. It was found that chlorine gas reacts with slaked lime to give a solid which retains the sanitizing and bleaching action of the chlorine, when it is mixed with water.

### Sodium Hypochlorite

Bleaching powder is inconvenient to use for many reasons. It is not very soluble in water and has to be used as a sort of slurry or "milk." The powder tends to lose its chlorine in a damp atmosphere, so the amount of chlorine in a sample can vary from almost the theoretical maximum to a very low figure, hardly enough to give any sanitizing effect at all. Such a material is obviously too variable to be acceptable for general use.

Chlorine is also absorbed by other alkalis than slaked lime, and with sodium hydroxide it gives *sodium hypochlorite,* sometimes known as eau de Javelle. Sodium hypochlorite is a solid, but it has only rarely been prepared in this form; normally it is sold as a solution in water, slightly yellow in color and having a strong characteristic smell, rather like chlorine gas but sharper. It has a biting taste because of its damaging effect on the tongue, but in low concentrations it tastes like chlorine water. At all concentrations, sodium hypochlorite tends to decompose into sodium chloride (common salt) and oxygen gas.

The oxygen originally appears in the "active" form also produced by chlorine gas, but if there is no organic material present to be oxidized, the oxygen comes off as gas. Above about 15 per cent sodium hypochlorite, this evolution of oxygen becomes so rapid that the product must not be kept in a closed container, and retains its effectiveness for only a few days: accordingly, this level is about the most concentrated that is normally manufactured or supplied. Even below this concentration, the hypochlorite gives off a steady stream of oxygen, and suppliers normally fit their containers with vented caps or some similar device to prevent a build-up of pressure.

This steady decomposition means that the strength of a sample of hypochlorite will steadily diminish as it is stored. It becomes necessary therefore to have some universal analytical convention for declaring the amount of active material in a sample when it leaves the supplier, and also so that the user can be sure of having enough active material to bleach, sanitize, or whatever other action is required. As the activity of sodium hypochlorite, and all the other chlorinating agents we shall consider, depends on the amount of active oxygen they will produce in water, and this in turn depends on the amount of chlorine gas they could theoretically produce, it is normal to declare the strength of such substances in terms of "available chlorine." This is the amount of chlorine gas they would theoretically produce if entirely hydrolyzed. The highest concentration of hypochlorite which it is safe to package contains about 14 per cent available chlorine, and this is normally the strength of the product supplied in bulk by the primary manufacturers. The breakdown of this material is still rather rapid for purposes of sale in smaller units, where the packs may be kept for weeks in a depot or store, and then kept for a further time by the customer, so suppliers usually dilute the hypochlorite still further. Ten per cent average available chlorine is common in the better products, while some of the cheaper ones may contain as little as 3-4 per cent. At this end of the scale, the production of oxygen is so slight that the products are sometimes packed in unvented containers.

For general maintenance work, the 14 per cent material, though theoretically cheaper per pound of chlorine purchased, will probably be found uneconomical in practice. It is usually only available in bulk packs, and by the time the user has disposed of 10-20 gallons, the strength may well have dropped to 10 per cent or less. Very dilute hypochlorite, 3-4 per cent, is cheaper per gallon, but after the extra cost of packaging has been considered, it is probably most ecomonical to buy hypochlorite in the 8-10 per cent range. This has a shelf-life of several weeks, is available in convenient packages, and is quite strong enough for any purposes of maintenance work.

Hypochlorite, considered as a germicide, will obviously be used in conjunction with other products, detergents and so on. It would be very desirable for mixtures of hypochlorite and detergent to be commercially available, but unfortunately this brings up the major disadvantage of the product. It is so reactive that it attacks *all* organic matter, and this includes soap, detergents, other germicides, etc. A mixture of liquid detergent and hypochlorite can be made, using nonionic or anionic detergents, and such a mixture makes an excellent germicidal cleanser, but after about 12 hours the detergent will have been destroyed, and the hypochlorite converted to simple sodium chloride solution. The same principle applies to mixtures of hypochlorite with most other cleansing or disinfecting material. The user can make these up for the occasion, but they do not keep, and suppliers have not yet solved the problem of making them do so, despite a great deal of research.

Hypochlorite should *never* be mixed with acid materials (this produces chlorine gas very quickly, and at least one laboratory worker has lost her life through a mistake of this kind), and in particular, it should not be mixed with acid powder toilet cleansers. Hypochlorite mixed with detergents or other cleansers should *never* be kept in a closed container. All these mixtures give off oxygen, and if the detergents contain urea or ammonium salts, there may be a rapid and dangerous evolution of nitrogen gas, producing a hazardous pressure in the bottle or can. Even if the container does not explode, there is a danger that liquid will be splashed up into the operator's face as the container is opened.

Hypochlorite should not be used as a germicide on wool, silk, nylon, colored materials (unless they are known to be fast to chlorine), or melamine tableware. This last prohibition is not because of the dangers of gross damage, but because chlorine is absorbed by this type of plastic and produces a very odd taste in coffee or other drinks placed in the cups afterwards.

With these limitations, sodium hypochlorite is a most useful and versatile germicide, economical in use (about 1/10 fluid ounce per gallon of water, using the 10 per cent available chlorine solution, is quite enough for nearly all germicidal purposes), and sure in its results. As far as is known, hypochlorite in sufficient quantity will kill any micro-organism.

Some recommendations for the use of hypochlorite and other chlorinating agents may refer to "Parts per million of available chlorine." The calculation is simple if the percentage of available chlorine is known. For example, if the hypochlorite purchased is 10 per cent available chlorine, and the recommendation is for 40 parts per million (p.p.m.), then 400 p.p.m. of the hypochlorite will be needed, or one part in 2500 parts of water. This is one fluid ounce of hypochlorite in 2500 fluid ounces of water, or 156¼ pints of water, or about 1/20 fluid ounce per gallon.

*Chloramine T.* The fact that sodium hypochlorite cannot be mixed with other cleansing materials for salable products has led to interest in various other chlorinating agents that are in solid form, and can therefore be mixed with other solid ingredients without any loss of chlorine until the mixture is dissolved in water. One of these solid materials is Chloramine T (sodium paratoluene-sulfo-chloramide), which contains about 25 per cent available chlorine. The chlorine is quite stable in the solid material, and therefore mixtures with detergent powders, etc., can be made. As soon as the powder is dissolved in water, Chloramine T releases its chlorine, which can then act as a germicide in the normal way.

*Dichloramine T* is a closely related compound containing two atoms of chlorine per molecule, and an available chlorine level of around 58 per cent. It is not nearly as soluble in water as Chloramine T, but finds use in antiseptic sprays and similar compounds.

*Chlorinated sodium phosphate* (chlorinated trisodium phosphate, sodium orthophosphate hypochlorite) is a crystalline mixture of trisodium phosphate, a very alkaline salt, and sodium hypochlorite. It is reasonably stable, but tends to lose chlorine when exposed to moisture. The normal commercial material contains about 3 per cent of available chlorine.

Chlorinated sodium phosphate is used in many alkaline cleansers, such as dairy sterilizers, machine dishwashing powders, and products of this kind, where the alkalinity of the phosphate is also essential for the cleansing action. It is an expensive way to buy active chlorine, but if the formulation requires alkali as well then the ready-made mixture may be useful.

## Isocyanurates

Derivatives of isocyanuric acid can be prepared containing up to three atoms of active chlorine per molecule. Two of these are widely used as sources of chlorine. *Trichloroisocyanuric acid* (TCCA) contains about 87 per cent of available chlorine (theoretically about 89 per cent, but the commercial material is not quite pure) and is probably the cheapest source of available chlorine except the gas itself, considering the price per pound of chlorine yielded. It is widely used as a bleach and sterilizer in scouring powders and machine dishwashing powders; care must be exercised in its use because it is very reactive and corrosive in the concentrated form. *Sodium dichloroisocyanurate* (NaDCCA or DCCA) is a similar compound, containing about 57 per cent available chlorine (theoretically nearly 63 per cent) and rather more stable than TCCA. At present costs, its available chlorine is more expensive than from TCCA, but it can be used for all the same purposes.

*Halazone* (Pantocide, para-carboxyphenyl-sulfodichloramide) is a very stable powder containing about 25 per cent available chlorine. It is used extensively compressed into tablets for sterilizing water supplies on the small scale or in emergencies.

*Chloro-hydantoin* is similar in its properties to TCCA. It contains about 50 per cent of available chlorine (theoretically 52 per cent).

All these solid chlorinating agents have the same properties towards micro-organisms as the equivalent amount of chlorine gas or sodium hypochlorite. They also have the same limitations, and should not be used on wool, silk, or colored goods, etc., without the same precautions as for sodium hypochlorite.

IODINE

Iodine is closely related, chemically, to chlorine, and has very similar properties in contact with micro-organisms; it destroys bacteria, molds, yeasts and viruses. It is also reactive with other organic materials, and will attack proteins such as wool and silk. As it is highly colored itself, and tends to stain other materials brown, its usefulness is limited.

Iodine is not very soluble in water but it is soluble in alcohol and solutions of potassium iodide, so one of these is usually employed to prepare antiseptic solutions of the material. *Lugol's solution* is a concentrated iodine solution containing 5 per cent iodine in a 10 per cent solution of potassium iodide. It is mainly used for internal purposes (the treatment of iodine deficiency, or for thyrotoxicosis) but it can also be used as a reliable reservoir compound with plenty of available iodine. *Tincture of iodine* as used for cuts and bruises is 2.5 per cent of iodine and 2.5 per cent of potassium iodide in a mainly alcoholic solution.

Iodine can be absorbed into loose chemical compounds with several materials, including polyvinylpyrrolidone (PVP), a soluble plastic material used as a base for hair lacquers and as a synthetic blood plasma substitute, and various polyethylene glycols—water-soluble waxy materials related to the polyethylene glycol type nonionic detergents. These compounds are non-staining and less reactive than ordinary iodine preparations, but they seem to release their iodine slowly in an active form that retains its germicidal action. The compounds are known collectively as *iodophors,* and they are effective against all types of micro-organisms.

FORMALDEHYDE

Formaldehyde is a colorless gas with an irritant smell. It dissolves readily in water, and is usually supplied in the form of a 36 to 40 per cent solution called *formalin.* Formaldehyde is a general protoplasmic poison, and kills bacteria, molds, yeasts and viruses; it is widely used as a sterilizing and preservative agent in medical and biological work. It has, however, several disadvantages as a product for general hygiene: its odor is penetrating and irritating, it causes dermatitis when in contact with the skin of many people, and it tends to be so reactive that it combines chemically with many of the materials that might be used in cleaning products, thus altering their characteristics and losing its own germicidal powers. Its use is therefore restricted to large-scale fumigation and similar operations. It is not really suitable for incorporation in general cleaning products.

There are several compounds of formaldehyde that release the gas slowly, and can therefore be used as germicides. Such materials are the *methylol-melamines* and *methylol-hydantoins*. So far they have not found much use in general cleaning and hygiene, but they have, like formaldehyde itself, very great germicidal activity against a wide range of organisms.

ETHYLENE OXIDE

This is a highly reactive gas, flammable and irritating. Like formaldehyde, it is a general protoplasmic poison, and kills all types of micro-organisms. It is used for sterilizing and fumigating the holds of ships, etc., where its gaseous form is a great advantage for penetration of the whole of the space.

## TYPES OF GERMICIDAL PRODUCTS

It will have been obvious that the various types of germicides all have their strengths and weaknesses, and the formulator of products must take account of these when trying to make his formulas effective, economical, and pleasant to use (as well as the other features automatically expected in product development—stable, non-corrosive and cheap). It is wasteful and dangerous to include, say, a cationic germicide in a product containing polyphosphates or an anionic detergent. Wasteful because a valuable germicide will be entirely inactivated by this treatment, and dangerous because users may rely on the product to carry out its germicidal promise merely because it contains the claimed germicide. The following notes, therefore, are intended to indicate the most suitable types of germicide for various types of products.

### Dishwashing Detergents

Dishwashing is carried out with a fairly low concentration of detergent in the presence of a very large amount of soiling, so that any germicide used must be effective under these adverse conditions. Phenols and chlorinated phenols are eliminated altogether because of their strong odor and taste, which would immediately taint dishes. Complex phenols and related compounds are too expensive and not effective enough against the chief "kitchen" organisms. The best germicides for dishwashing are chlorine derivatives or cationic germicides.

Chlorine has the advantage that it is very effective at low concentrations, and can deal not only with bacteria but molds and yeasts. It can be added in two ways: sodium hypochlorite solution can be used in conjunction with a conventional liquid detergent, or a solid chlorine source such as trichloroisocyanuric acid or Chloramine T can be added to a powder detergent. The former method, of course, requires that the hypochlorite is added only shortly before use, as the mixtures will be unstable and will not keep more than about 12 hours (the hypochlorite decomposes the detergent slowly and is itself decomposed in the process). Either liquid hypochlorite can be added to an equal amount of liquid detergent at the beginning of the day's work, or the two liquids can be dosed into the sink together by means of a double venturi tap proportioner (see next chapter for details of these devices). In either case, a solution of equal parts of 10 per cent hypochlorite, mixed with a 25 per cent active detergent liquid used at 1/8 ounce per gallon, will give reasonable cleansing and about 50 p.p.m. active chlorine in the dishwashing water.

The powders containing solid chlorinating agents can be used in a similar way; as long as they are kept dry, the chlorine will not affect the other ingredients.

The great disadvantage of chlorine in dishwashing is its smell; in the presence of some food residues, notably fat, this seems to become even more pronounced. It also discolors cutlery of all kinds, even stainless steel. Cationic germicides are free from these troubles, as they are usually almost odorless and have no staining effect. Unfortunately they cannot be mixed with the commonest type of dishwashing detergent, the anionic type, without inactivation of germicidal *and* detergent powers. They must therefore be mixed with nonionic detergents, which are more expensive and give less foam than the anionic type. The final product is therefore more costly and appears in the dishwasher's eyes to be less efficient than the conventional anionic dishwashing compound. However, if the actual cleaning powers of such a combination are judged by results, not by lather, the germicidal product will prove itself. A product containing about 8-10 per cent of nonionic detergent of the nonylphenol condensate type, and 6 per cent of benzalkonium chloride (@ 100 per cent—12 per cent of the commercial product) or a similar cationic germicide, is an effective dishwasher and sterilant at levels around 1/5 ounce per gallon. Such a product can give kills of the order of 99+ per cent against organisms like *Staphylococcus albus* and *Escherichia coli* under dishwashing conditions.

## Scourers

Because of the combined germicidal and stain-removing effect, the chlorine sources are best for addition to scourers. Sodium dichloroisocyanurate or trichloroisocyanuric acid at a level suitable to give 1-2 per cent of active chlorine in the powder will achieve a marked germicidal effect. This will be assisted by the fact that the powders are usually used at high concentrations, often being made up as a thick paste with very little water, so that the chlorine available at the surface of vessels may be at a level of 1000 p.p.m. or more.

There have been suggestions for using Vancide BN and similar germicides in scouring powders, but the stain-removing powers and cheapness of chlorinating agents have secured priority for these at present.

## Laundry Detergents

While the addition of a suitable germicide to laundry detergents would be of some benefit, not very much has been done in this direction as yet. One very useful process in laundry work, however, is to use cationic germicides in the rinse stage of fabric washing, so that the germicidal effect is retained after drying.

Cationic germicides as a class are very strongly attracted to surfaces, such as those of cotton goods, and even more strongly to proteins, such as wool, and polyamides, such as nylon. On the surface they remain firmly fixed, even through the rinsing stages, and impart to the surface not only germicidal or bacteriostatic properties but a soft "handle" as well. This is the basis of the rinse products and softeners, and similar materials used in the rinse stage.

Proprietary softeners tend to concentrate on the feel of the fabric at the expense of the germicidal power of the product, but very good results can be obtained in both senses by adding a small amount of benzalkonium chloride or cetrimide to the final rinse of woolens, babies' diapers, towels, and similar goods. The application to diapers can be particularly useful, as the germicide retained on the material kills the bacteria that would otherwise break down urine into ammonia, which causes diaper rash. A solution of 0.1 per cent benzalkonium chloride is suitable for this purpose.

Blankets can also be treated in this way, and a 0.1 per cent benzalkonium chloride solution will kill most of the bacteria on blankets if used as the last rinse, and at the same time keep the material soft. For hospital use, or in other circumstances where it is important to reduce the bacterial population to a minimum, higher concentrations will be necessary, as such organisms as *Streptococcus pyogenes* and *Pseudomonas aeruginosa* can survive 0.1 per cent benzalkonium chloride.

## Carpet Shampoos

Germicides may be added to carpet shampoos to cut down the resident population of bacteria in the carpet, to prevent the spread of bacteria during the vacuuming stage, and to impart to the carpet some semi-permanent bacteriostatic property. The germicide must be selected with care, as chlorinating agents would harm the wool and perhaps the color of the carpet, and if the normal high-foaming anionic carpet shampoo materials are used, cationic germicides are ruled out because of imcompatibility. The best type of germicide to use is one of the complex phenols, such as Vancide BN at about 0.25 per cent in the conventional shampoo detergent at about 10 per cent active detergent.

It should be understood that the residual germicide on the carpet cannot kill bacteria when the carpet is dry, but only when it is wet.

## Floor Polishes

The addition of a germicide to the conventional acrylic type of dry-bright polish will help to maintain hygiene in areas where harmful bacteria may well be spread by traffic across the floor. As long as the polish is formulated to avoid polyanions, the best type of germicide is undoubtedly a cationic one, preferably chlorhexidine, which has a wider range of germicidal activity than most of the other cationics; use at about 0.1 per cent in the normal polish is satisfactory.

Alternatively, a complex phenol of the Vancide type may be used at about 0.25 per cent. In either case, there will be residual germicidal activity from the germicide left in the polish, and this activity will be revived when the floor is re-wetted for cleaning.

When applying a germicidal polish, it is good practice to strip any old polish from the floor beforehand. Not only will the old polish retain dirt, but it may contain ingredients which are incompatible with the germicides in the new polish.

## General Sanitizers

There is a considerable market for general sanitizers to be added to cleaning solutions. It may be helpful to recapitulate the main types.

*Black fluids* are essentially crude coal-tar phenol or cresol; they are dark, oily, strong-smelling, poisonous, and generally unpleasant, and have been superseded for all practical purposes by the more refined types.

*White fluids* are emulsions of better-grade cresol in soap solution, also known as Lysol. They are effective, but rather strong smelling and distinctly poisonous. As a cheap all-purpose sanitizer the white fluid is economically attractive, but precautions should be taken when handling the materials.

*Chlorinated phenol* sanitizers are made from PCMX or DCMX in similar soap emulsion; they are much less poisonous than Lysol but have similar sanitizing powers. PCMX can be obtained in a number of commercial grades, from brown oily material to pure white crystals. The products made from these obviously reflect the standard of the germicide. Usually the better grades are used in antiseptics and the poorer ones in household sanitizers.

*Pine oil* sanitizers are made almost entirely of pine oil, and thus contain mainly turpentine-like material plus resins. They are not very effective.

*Pine* sanitizers, which are often sold, may be confused with the last type, but are really chlorinated phenol sanitizers with a small amount of pine perfume added to cover up unpleasant smells. They have the same limitations as the chlorinated phenol types.

*Cationic* sanitizers have not had a great success on the general market, perhaps because they do not turn cloudy in water as do the phenolics, and they do not have the "sanitizer odor" of the chlorinated phenols. However, particularly for general antiseptic use, they are far superior to the phenolics.

## Aerosol Sprays

There is a market for germicidal preparations in the form of aerosol sprays which can be directed over any surface or object that is believed to be unhygienic. This development must be regarded with some caution, as there are two reasons why it is unlikely that such products can be effective. First, it is clear that not much of the solution can be used at a time, and therefore the solution must be concentrated. If this is the case, the fine aerosol spray is likely to lose all its water by evaporation before it reaches the surface, and there are no germicides except the gases ethylene oxide and formaldehyde that can kill bacteria in the dry state. They all need water. The other objection is that the spray cannot remove soiling, not even as much as the casual wipe with a sponge or cloth dipped in sanitizer, and therefore soiling material will be left to protect the bacteria and perhaps even act as nutrient for them.

In general, these products seem likely to cause a false feeling of confidence, unsupported by any real reduction in the bacterial population.

# five

# Tools and Machines

In the previous chapters, we have considered in detail the products used in cleaning various surfaces and articles. Equally important for an efficient cleaning job is mechanical action, and rubbing, scouring, brushing, scarifying, polishing, buffing and dusting are only some of the mechanical activities used in cleaning and maintenance. Many articles and surfaces can be cleaned, at least partially, by mechanical action alone, as in vacuum cleaning and vacuum sweeping, and in general the more work applied to a cleaning process, the less cleaning product that is needed.

The human hand, so versatile in general and capable of many mechanical uses, is a very poor cleaning device. It is relatively small, irregularly shaped, does not hold water well, and is likely to be damaged by friction far more easily than most of the surfaces with which it comes into contact. It is not surprising, therefore, that men have extended the cleaning action of the hand with various tools from the dawn of history; Homer describes Penelope's servants washing down tables with sponges before a meal. Pliny mentions the use in ancient Rome of sponges fastened to poles as mops, an idea that seems to have been forgotten for centuries and then revived in modern times.

In this chapter the *tools,* i.e. simple extensions of the hand, will be considered first and then the *machines,* where electrical or other power is used to increase the efficiency of the cleaning process and to eliminate some or all of the manual labor.

## BRUSHES, MOPS, SQUEEGEES, ETC.

BRUSHES

A brush or broom is designed to remove dirt from surfaces without the use of water, either as the total process, or to remove coarse surface dirt before washing. The bristles of a broom should be firm enough to have a chisel-like action on dirt which is slightly adherent to the surface, such as a light deposit of mud or slightly sticky refuse, prizing it off the ground and keeping it moving, but they must also be flexible enough to remain in contact with an irregular surface, and not so stiff or sharp that they damage the surface itself. General-purpose brooms are made of bristle, horsehair and bristle, nylon, tampico fiber with a casing of horsehair to give the necessary chisel action, or similar mixtures. For heavy-duty use, such as exterior concrete surfaces, whalebone may be added in the center of the head.

Sweeping should always be done slowly and deliberately—quick short jabs at the ground send more dust flying into the air than along the floor—and it is important to use the widest brush head consonant with reasonable weight and maneuverability. Even when properly done, however, sweeping is a very inefficient process, because more time and effort is spent moving the dirt along than actually dislodging it from the surface. For any but the smallest premises, the maintenance manager would do well to calculate the real cost of hand sweeping versus that of a suitable vacuum sweeper.

## MOPS

Mops are designed to carry water or other cleansing liquids and finishing fluids to a surface. The traditional mop is woven of soft cotton in fairly thick strands, in sizes varying from 8 ounces to 36 ounces. The weight of a 36-ounce mop head filled with water or detergent solution is considerable, especially at the end of the mop handle, and the 8-12 ounce range is most popular with female labor, the 20-24 ounce range for men. The old-fashioned methods of fastening mops to poles with a nail or rivet has entirely given place, in industry, to the use of quick release clamps. These are not only better for quick changing of mop heads, but they also encourage a greater degree of hygiene because the mop heads can be taken out for washing more efficiently and quickly.

Cotton mops, in common with other types, have to be squeezed out during use, to remove dirty water and to give the mop head greater powers of water pickup during the drying stage. The traditional mop pail with a perforated cone at the top, into which the mop head is pressed, is some improvement on squeezing out by hand, but not very much improvement, and every user of a mop should be given a suitable mechanical wringer on the bucket or bucket holder. Wringers are usually of the gear or flat-press type, and very efficient devices of this kind are available from Geerpress Wringer Inc. and the White Mop Wringer Co. who also have a full range of mop handles with clamps, buckets, and tanks, complete with trucks to carry two or more buckets for heavy jobs. It should be remembered that the efficiency of the mopping operation depends almost entirely on the efficiency of the wringing method, and deficiencies in this part of the equipment can increase the time taken quite alarmingly.

Considered as a physical system, a mop head in contact with a wet floor is a complex of forces. Capillary action attracts water up the fibers of the mop, and capillary action also tends to keep water on the floor. However, as the effective surface area of the mop head is very much greater than that of the floor immediately underneath it, the mop takes up by far the greater proportion of the liquid. It goes on soaking up water until the weight of water in the mop exerts a downward force equal to the upward force of the capillary attraction, and at this stage the mop head is saturated and will not pick up any more liquid. However, the important point is that, at any time between putting a dry mop on the floor and the point of saturation, the *rate* of pick-up of water is proportional to the difference between the capillary attraction and the weight of water already absorbed. The process, in mathematicians' jargon, is an *exponential* one, and in practice, if a mop head can hold, say, a maximum of one pint of water, starting from the completely dry state, and it soaks up a quarter of a pint of water in five seconds, it will take *ten* seconds to soak up the next quarter of a pint and *twenty* seconds to soak up a third quarter of a pint. Obviously if the mop head were left in contact with the water for an indefinite time it would not matter very much how long it took to soak up the water, but mops are usually passed over the floor rapidly, and no allowance is made for their degree of saturation. In consequence, a mop head that can be wrung out every time to, say, one-quarter of its saturated capacity, will soak up water four times as fast as a mop head that is only wrung out to three quarters of its saturated capacity, apart from any question of the number of passes necessary.

Similar considerations apply to sponge mops: some of the forces that lift water off a floor into a sponge are vacuum effects of narrow tubes in the sponge that have the air squeezed out of them against the floor, and take up water to replace the air as they are allowed to swell up again. The mathematics is the same, however. Many devices are on the market for squeezing sponge mops efficiently, and it is very well worthwhile to search for a really effective one.

The sponges used in these sponge mops are of two main types: cellulose sponges and polyurethane sponges. The cellulose type is usually pale brown, with fairly large irregular holes, and very stiff when dry. They should not be bent or squeezed in the dry state, or they may crack, and they should be wetted before they are fitted into holders. The sponges are strong and long-wearing, but like all cellulose materials they are subject to bacterial attack, and may rot if left wet for too long. If possible they should be rinsed out with a dilute solution of germicide—sodium hypochlorite at about 1/10 ounce of the 10 per cent active chlorine material per gallon would be quite suitable—and allowed to dry. Soap, if used, should not be allowed to dry in these sponges, otherwise the bacterial attack will be enhanced and an unpleasant slime produced in the interior of the sponge.

Polyurethane sponges are usually more evenly spaced with small holes, can be almost any color, and are soft even when dry. They are not nearly as hard wearing as cellulose sponges, but are not affected much by bacteria. They should not be used with sodium hypochlorite except in very low concentrations. Polyurethane sponges, because of their even construction and relative weakness, are better as applicators for liquid polish, etc., while cellulose sponges are better for cleansing.

SQUEEGEES

Squeegees, rubber blades held in a suitable horizontal grip, are often seen in window cleaning practice, and also have many applications for floors and other surfaces, particularly when there is a drain within easy access. The great advantage of the squeegee over the mop is that the mop can only "share" the water between itself and the floor: the mop takes the largest share, but there is always some moisture left on the surface, and this can dry to a streaky appearance if there is detergent or dirt still in the solution. With a squeegee, it is possible to leave a surface quite clean. On the other hand, the squeegee is useless on an irregular surface. Squeegees *can* be obtained in straight or curved shapes to meet specialized needs.

## Abrasive Pads

For many of the types of dirt that mopping alone cannot move, a mild abrasive is necessary. Scouring powder or scouring blocks used to be the main products for this purpose, but they have the disadvantage of leaving white deposits which have to be removed after the scouring is completed. More recently, scouring pads have been introduced, both for hand and machine use, which consist of a mat of non-woven plastic fiber, usually nylon, rather like a very open felt material, which has been dusted over with abrasive powder, such as fine aluminum oxide carborundum, and then exposed to just enough heat to melt the fiber very slightly. This heating has two effects: it melts the surface of the fiber enough for the abrasive to sink in and become firmly attached but still presents an abrasive surface, and it melts together the crossing points of the fibers, thus consolidating the fabric. These pads are very useful for most scouring purposes, as the abrasive rarely comes away from the pad, and the small pieces of fiber that wear off do not show up to the same extent as scouring powder residues. The felt is sufficiently absorbent to hold detergent solution or water, but it can also be attached to cellulose or polyurethane sponges. Scouring pads should not be used to any extent with sodium hypochlorite solutions, as these tend to decompose the nylon. If it is necessary to decontaminate them, boiling is the best way.

## TAP PROPORTIONERS

Liquid detergents, sanitizers, hypochlorite and other liquid materials are usually bought in fairly large containers—1-gallon, 2-gallon, and 5-gallon cans are common—for convenience in storage and economy in packaging material. Since they are used in small quantities, often as little as 1/10 ounce at a time, the questions arise, how to insure that the products are not wasted in the process of pouring them from the large container, and how to make sure that operators do not use too much product in their cleaning work. Spilling or pilferage from the can during dispensing can quickly lead to major losses, but possibly even more material is lost by constant overuse of the product. Obviously a 2- or 5-gallon can is too unwieldy to be handled near a sink for pouring, and most people will use an intermediate vessel, such as a jar or a household detergent pack that has been refilled from the can.

These compromises are not really satisfactory because they do not prevent anyone from tipping an ounce of liquid into a bucket of water when only one tenth of that quantity may be needed. Tap proportioners are the solution to this problem. They are devices that can be fitted to a water tap, and will dose in detergent, sanitizer or bleach at will, in quantities previously calculated as being best for the type of cleaning carried out in the premises.

A typical proportioner design is shown in Figure 5.1b, which is a diagrammatic section. The principle is essentially that of the venturi: if water flows through a tube with a restriction in its length, as at A in Figure 5.1a, there will be a lowering or pressure at the restriction, and if a side tube is fitted at this point, the lowered pressure will create suction in the side tube. Air or liquid from the side tube will be sucked into the stream of water through the main tube, and the quantities taken in will increase as the speed of flow in the main tube increases. Such a system is

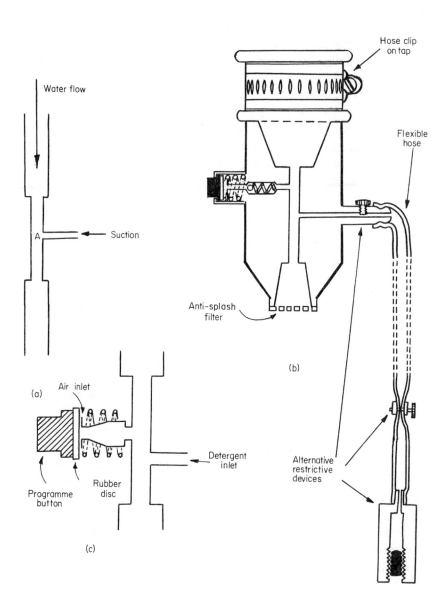

Figure 5.1

(a) Venturi principle. (b) Diagrammatic section of tap proportioner. The various restrictive devices shown on the detergent inlet are alternative methods, and would not be used together. (c) Details of detergent control by opening or closing air inlet, using the programming button.

called a *venturi,* after the inventor, and the idea is used in many hydraulic systems and also as a means of measuring the speed of water or other liquids passing along a pipe.

In a tap proportioner, the main stream of water comes from a tap and the side tube leads, via a flexible pipe, to a can of detergent or other cleansing liquid. This reservoir must be kept below the level of the tap, otherwise detergent, once sucked into the system, would siphon through continuously; most people put the can under the sink or in some similar place on the floor. As long as there is a sufficient flow of water from the tap to generate suction enough to lift the liquid from the level of the detergent can to the height of the side tube, liquid will be fed into the main stream of water.

Obviously two controls are necessary. It must be possible to govern the rate of addition of the detergent or other liquid so as to give the required dosage. This is done by restricting the side tube in various ways, either a small screw that reduces the effective cross section of the side tube, a screw clip that compresses the flexible tube or restrictive devices that fit on the lower end of the flexible tube. Such devices vary from one manufacturer to another; the essentials of any such device are that it should be easy to adjust it to fine limits by *authorized* users, but not so easy that cleaning staff can meddle with it. All three types of devices are shown in Figure 5.1b. The fitting at the bottom of the flexible tube is essentially a threaded tube, which has a small threaded plug screwed into it. The thread on the plug is slightly "topped" by rubbing down the threads, so that it does not exactly fit the internal thread of the outer tube but leaves a fine helical capillary tube running along the thread. This acts as a very long capillary that can be shortened by unscrewing the plug a little, or lengthened by screwing it further in; such a device gives very accurate control over the entry of liquid.

The second control necessary is a means of switching off the detergent supply altogether so that plain water can be obtained from the tap. This could be done by having a constricting device that cuts off the detergent supply altogether, but any failure of this would mean leakage of detergent when it was not wanted. In practice the most popular on/off control is a *second* side-tube leading to the air. When this is open, air is sucked into the water-stream and liquid detergent is not, because all the suction naturally acts on the easiest "fluid," the air. If the air inlet is closed by pressing the control button, a plate covers the air inlet tube, and all the suction is applied to the detergent: in addition, the suction holds the plate down over the air inlet tube. This method has a "fail-safe" feature in that as soon as the tap is turned off, the suction ceases and the plate over the air inlet is returned by a light spring so that the air inlet is opened again. Next time the tap is turned on, no detergent will be taken up until the control button is pressed again. This prevents unwanted contamination of water by detergent. Figure 5.1c illustrates the action of the program button.

Two other refinements should be mentioned:

1. All tap proportioners should have a non-return valve fitted to the detergent inlet tube; otherwise, when the tap is turned off and suction ceases, the detergent will gradually sink back down the flexible tube to the level of the liquid in the can, and if the pipe is a long one it may take several minutes to suck the liquid all the way back next time it is needed.

2. All tap proportioners should have some means of cutting off the supply of detergent slightly before the flow of water ceases. This is to ensure that the proportioner is not left with traces of detergent inside, which could be washed out into water which was required free of detergent for cooking or drinking. There are various patented devices for making sure that the last drops of detergent are swilled out by the last flow of water as the tap is turned off.

Tap proportioners, especially if run from hot taps, may become furred up with water hardness salts to such an extent that they cease to act properly or at all. The manufacturers usually offer servicing at set periods, but if this is not available, the best treatment is to take the proportioner off the tap, remove any loose scale and dirt by brushing with a bottle brush or old toothbrush, and then immerse the whole device in a solution of sodium dihydrogen phosphate (3 ounces to a pint of water) until the scale is removed. Proprietary products for descaling auto radiators can also be used; they are of course more expensive than buying the phosphate as such. As far as possible, avoid poking anything down the venturi; the proportioners are made to quite fine degrees of accuracy, and may be damaged by such treatment.

The simplest way of regulating the dosage to a tap proportioner is to obtain a bucket of known capacity, say 2 gallons, and a small measuring cylinder or other graduated measure with markings in cubic centimeters; the accuracy is not very important. Place the measuring cylinder on the floor where the detergent can is going to stand, fill the cylinder with detergent, noting the level, and then place the detergent inlet tube of the proportioner in the cylinder. Turn the tap on to give a reasonable flow of water and press the "on" button, with a bucket under the tap. When the bucket is filled with detergent solution, note the new level of detergent in the measuring cylinder.

If the required dosage is, say, 1/5 ounce of detergent per gallon, and the bucket 2 gallons, the consumption of detergent should be about 12 cubic centimeters. If it is more than this, reduce the detergent flow a little; if less, open up a little, and then repeat the measurement, adjusting until the dosage is correct.

It will be found impossible to adjust the dosage with great accuracy, because, unfortunately, the intake of detergent is not exactly proportional to the flow of water. In fact, the pressure difference at the restriction, and hence the suction, is proportional to the *square* of the speed of water flow. A tap that is delivering 2 gallons per minute and sucking up 1/2 ounce of detergent per minute will suck up 2 ounces of detergent per minute if it is turned on to give 4 gallons of water per minute. The dosage in the first case is 1/4 ounce per gallon, but doubling the rate of flow brings it to 1/2 ounce per gallon. The best arrangement, unless the flow from the tap is very fast, is to turn it on full for the dosage adjustment, and err a little on the side of generosity in fixing the dosage under these conditions.

Tap proportioners can be used for liquid detergents or sanitizers. For sodium hypochlorite, because of the low viscosity of the liquid, a special inlet control is necessary, and the proportioner itself should be made of plastic or other non-corrodible materials such as stainless steel.

Some proportioners are supplied with two venturis and two control buttons and side tubes; these can be used for detergent and sanitizer combined.

Users should consult their water authority before fitting tap proportioners to taps that draw water directly from the mains; some of the devices on the market have faults in contruction which could lead to siphoning back of detergent solution into the water main. Taps supplied indirectly, from water tanks, do not produce this hazard.

## VACUUM CLEANERS

The machines to be considered in this section are those that remove dirt and other dry debris by sucking it up in a stream of air and then filtering the airstream so as to trap the dirt; the airstream has not only to remove the dirt, but has to produce sufficient mechanical action to dislodge it.

The user or prospective purchaser of such a machine should assess its operation primarily at three stages, which represent the main efficiency criteria:

1. Can suction really be directed exactly where it is needed? Are there sufficient means of extension, are the nozzles and tools designed for the type of cleaning undertaken by the user, and will they penetrate to the most awkward

corners of the premises? Secondly, is the machine itself sufficiently portable for the type of labor and the layout of the building?

Obviously the right choice of machine must depend on the circumstances. In an old building with many stairs and small offices with many cramped corners, a machine weighing more than about 20 pounds will not be used efficiently (or at all, when the supervisor's back is turned). In a modern single-story factory with large areas of open floor, a very large machine may be quite satisfactory, and may indeed be the only one of sufficient size and power to be efficient.

2. Is the suction really powerful enough to dislodge dirt, as well as carrying it into the dust bag? A few calculations may throw a new light on the actual forces at work in vacuum cleaning. A good industrial vacuum cleaner will draw over 100 cubic feet of air per minute at its best (i.e. close to the machine and fitted with a wide orifice head; extensions and narrow heads tend to cut down the suction both by leakage and friction applied to the air by the walls of the tubes and nozzles. The Breuer Tornado 98700 suction unit, for example, an excellent high-power machine, draws 53 cubic feet per minute with a 3/4-inch orifice, but 144 cubic feet per minute with a 2-inch orifice). Let us assume an intermediate figure of 100 cubic feet per minute at the outlet, which is 6000 cubic feet per hour. This seems a large amount of air, but the flow velocity is also dependent on the cross-sectional area of the pipe. With the machine just quoted, 100 c.f.m. would be attained with a nozzle of about 1 1/4 inches diameter, or approximately 1 1/4 square inches area. The linear flow of air is therefore 130 miles per hour. If, however, the normal type of floor or carpet tool is fitted to this outlet nozzle, the area through which the air is drawn becomes much greater and the velocity drops. A 14-inch nozzle, 1/2 inch wide (and therefore 7 square inches area) will reduce the 130 miles per hour to about 23 miles per hour, about Beaufort 5 or a "moderate wind." Moderate winds can raise loose dust quite effectively, but they may not have very much effect on any dirt that is even slightly adhesive to the floor. It is important, then to choose a cleaner with ample power, and not to overrate the size of the tools that can be used.

3. Is the dust really trapped adequately before the air is released? A vacuum cleaner represents an attempt to reconcile two almost totally opposed requirements. At the nozzle end the airflow must be as fast and free as possible, while at the filter end the smallest particles must be trapped, which means using a filter that inevitably restricts the flow of air. If the filter is inadequate the surroundings of the cleaner will be showered with fine dust and bacteria, while if it is too restrictive the airflow at the nozzle will fall far short of the 100 cubic feet per minute that was quoted earlier.

Taking these three criteria in turn, the user can decide which is of most vital interest for his particular circumstances. Essentially, is portability, power, or filter efficiency the most important matter?

### Portability

A vacuum cleaner should not weigh more than about 20 pounds if it has to be lifted about, carried up stairs, and so on. Casters, wheels, or efficient runners should be fitted, or available as an attachment, to facilitate movement when the machine is used on the floor. Vacuum cleaners tend to have most of their weight concentrated in the motor and impeller, while the cylinder or dust bag is light, and therefore balance is as important an aspect of design as overall weight. Some extra-light machines are designed for use on the operator's back or otherwise.

**Table 5.1 Portable Vacuum Cleaners**

| Model | Motor power | Vacuum " water lift | CFM | Cord length | Weight |
|---|---|---|---|---|---|
| Hild Strap-Bak-Vac 750-¾ | ¾ HP | 52" | 225 | 30' | 14 lb. |
| Hild Strap-Bak-Vac 750-1½ | 1½ HP | 68" | 250 | 30' | 16 lb. |
| Nobles Strap-a-vac | | | 69.2 | 50' | 10 lb. |
| Clarke Napsac | 1 HP | | | 50' | 11½ lb. |
| General Floor-craft* Buddy-vac | 1 HP | 55" | | 40' | 12¼ lb. |
| Advance Papoose | 1 HP | 82" | | 40' | 10 lb. |
| Breuer Pac-vac | 7/8 -2 HP (3 units) | | | 25'-50' | Varies with motor unit |
| World Floor Wasp | 1 HP | 82" | | 40' | 10 lb. |

Most of these portable machines hold between 1/4 bushel and 1/3 bushel dry material. The measure of inches of "water-lift" is another characteristic of vacuum cleaners, sometimes quoted instead of or in addition to cubic feet of air per minute (CFM). The water-lift shows the vacuum power for raising water in a vertical tube: the higher the water lift, the better the vacuum.

Most of these machines can be carried both on the back and on a "dolly" or other carriage; some have "snap-on" wheels that can be fitted to the body. When carried on the back, these machines are particularly

*See Plate 1.

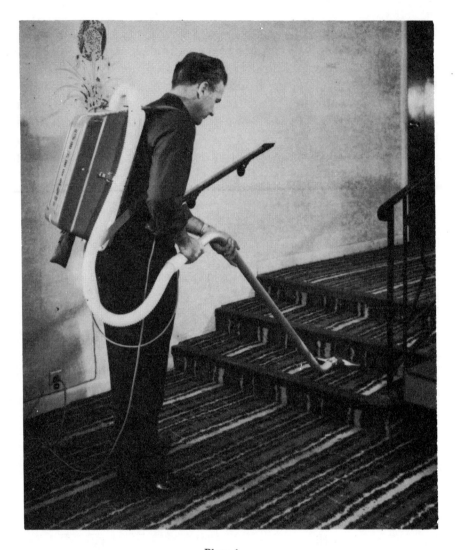

Plate 1
Buddy-Vac Portable Vacuum Cleaner (Courtesy of General Floorcraft Inc., 3630 Rombouts Ave., Bronx, New York, N.Y. 10466)

suited for high work, such as curtains, ledges, the tops of cupboards, light fixtures, and so on.

### Suction

While portable machines are quite adequate for all normal cleaning work, and the companies which supply them can also supply rather larger

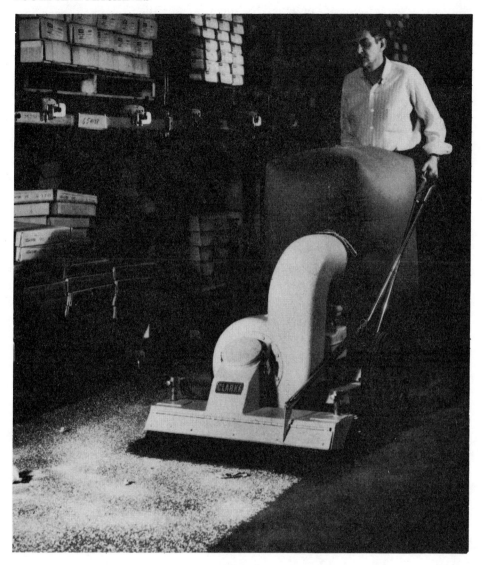

Plate 2
Clarke Litter-Vac (Courtesy of Clarke Floor Machine Company, 2800 Estes Street, Muskegon, Mich. 49443)

machines for ground-level work, there are obviously certain jobs which need a far larger nozzle, and therefore far more power if the suction is to be adequate. One of the most difficult problems is the removal of trash from large open spaces, such as waste paper from parks, car parking areas, theaters, schools and playgrounds, and sawdust, litter and sand from large engineering works and building sites. Large machines are marketed by several companies that will deal with this type of litter, even beer cans and similar large objects. Plate 2 shows a machine that will pick up any type of litter including paper plates and cups, metal washers, gravel, broken glass, metal chips, leaves, twigs (and damp vegetable waste; a special high-wet-strength bag is used for this purpose) and any similar materials that need to be removed or salvaged. Similar machines are listed in Table 5.2.

**Table 5.2 Large Vacuum Cleaners**

| Model | Power | CFM | Capacity | Weight |
|---|---|---|---|---|
| Advance Roamer 3 HP | 3 HP gas | | 5 cu. ft. | 87 lb. |
| Advance Roamer 5 HP | 5 HP gas | | 11 cu. ft. | 150 lb. |
| Advance Roamer 6HP | 6 HP gas or propane | | 11 cu. ft. | 150-200 lb. |
| Advance Electric Roamer | 1 HP | | 3 cu. ft. | 107 lb. |
| Advance Battery Roamer | 1 HP | | 7 cu. ft. | 184 lb. without batteries |
| Atlas Greyhound | 3HP cord electric | | 3 cu. ft. | 111 lb. |
| Clarke 580 Spacevac | 1 HP cord electric | 200 | 5 cu. ft. | 130 lb. |
| Clarke Litter Vac* | 4 HP gas | | 11 cu. ft. | 167 lb. |
| Billy Goat | 8 HP gas | | 12 cu. ft. | |
| National Super Service Grazer | 6 HP gas | | | 165 lb. |

## Filtration

Where the paramount need is for dust and bacteria to *stay* in the cleaner and not to be sprayed out in the exhaust air, it may be necessary to have quite a complex system of filters to achieve this. Premises such as hospitals, laboratories, and "white rooms" in factories therefore need a machine with a much better filter than the usual paper bag, and with facilities for inserting replaceable filters that will stop the passage of particles down to one micron (1/1000 millimeter). Such a filter is likely to

---

*See Plate 2.

cause a severe restriction to the airflow, and the power of the machine must be increased accordingly. A typical machine would have a conventional cloth filter that removes coarse particles and larger grains of dust, and then the air passes through the germicidal filter, a mass of polyurethane foam with more than 500,000 pores per cubic inch, which has been treated with a phenolic germicide. The filter contains 190 cubic inches of foam, or almost 100 million impregnated cells, and can stop particles down to 0.2 micron. In a test run where the machine was exposed to various bacteria, the number of bacteria escaping from the machine was reduced by the filter from 3,000 (without filter) to 18 (with treated filter) in unit time.

To "drive" such a complex system it is obvious that powerful suction must be employed. Most of the machines for which this system is recommended give a water-lift of 78 inches and contain 1 HP motors. Such powerful machines tend to be less portable than the simpler type, and again the weight range of machines in this power group is from 57-96 pounds.

## VACUUM SWEEPERS

Where the ordinary vacuum cleaners do not dislodge dirt sufficiently, it is necessary to use a cleaner with some means of mechanical action in addition to the airflow. In some household cleaners and some carpet machines rotary beaters are used, but the method of choice for large areas is brushing. With brushes to provide the force to dislodge dirt the suction does not have to be quite as powerful, but it is important that machines of this kind should have enough suction to prevent the dust raised by the brushes from being scattered about.

For cleaning large areas of carpet, a vacuum sweeper is undoubtedly the best type of machine. For example, using an efficient machine, 19,500 square feet of carpeting can be cleaned per hour, which would mean that all the carpeted areas of a very large hotel, for instance, could be cleaned during the hours when the public is not using the corridors and meeting rooms. Even larger machines are used for open spaces, including machines that can be ridden by the operator for sweeping roads and factory environs. Table 5.3 shows the wide range of vacuum sweepers available on the US market, from compact devices small enough to sweep carpets in narrow hallways to large outdoor sweepers.

It will be understood that all machines are powered by standard electricity from regular outlets unless otherwise stated. The larger machines usually have one or more side brooms to supplement the action of the

**Table 5.3 Vacuum Sweepers**

| Model | Brush width | Power (brush/vacuum) | Capacity | Weight |
|---|---|---|---|---|
| Hild Rug Pilelifter | 12" and 16" | ½ HP/¾ HP | | 68 lb. |
| Hild Rugavator 1113 | 13" | | | 49 lb. |
| Nobles Carpet-Vac | 13½" | 1/8 HP/1HP | ¼ cu. ft. | 45 lb. |
| Advance Carpetwin 14 | 14" | 1/8 HP/1HP | 1/3 cu. ft. | 35 lb. |
| Clarke 575 | 15¼" | 1/6HP/1HP | 1/3 cu. ft. | 45 lb. |
| General Flooring CM-1 | 15½" | 1/6 HP/1HP | 1/3 cu. ft. | 32 lb. |
| World Widget 140 | 18" | ¼HP/1HP | 2/3 cu. ft. | 56 lb. |
| Advance Carpetwin 20 | 20" | 1/8HP/1HP | 1/3 cu. ft. | 56 lb. |
| Tennant Carpet Cleaner | 21" | 1 HP | ½ cu. ft. | 125 lb. |
| World Wanderer 122 E | 22" | 1 HP | 2.2 cu. ft. | |
| Breuer Tornado Carpetkeeper | 22" | 5/8HP | | |
| American Lincoln A320 | 24" | 3 HP gas | 3 cu. ft. | 320 lb. |
| World Wanderer 126 E | 26" | 1 HP | 2.2 cu. ft. | |
| World Wanderer 126 G | 26" | 3 HP gas | 2.2 cu. ft. | |
| Advance Turbulator 30 | 30" | ¼HP/1¼HP | 1½ cu. ft. | 125 lb. |
| American Lincoln A 323 | 32" (with side broom) | 3 HP gas | 3 cu. ft. | 370 lb. |
| World Wanderer 134B | 34" | 0.8 HP (battery) | 7 cu. ft. | |
| World Wanderer 634G | 34" | 6 HP gas | 11 cu. ft. | |
| American Lincoln A330 | 36" | 5 HP gas | 5 cu. ft. | 430 lb. |

**Table 5.3 (cont.)**

| Model | Brush width | Power (brush/vacuum) | Capacity | Weight |
|---|---|---|---|---|
| American Lincoln A 1430 | 36" | 9.2 HP gas | 9 cu. ft. | 1300 lb. (ride) |
| Somerset 34 | 26" + 17" side | 1½ HP (battery) | 2½ cu.ft. | 304 lb. (without batteries) |
| Tennant 42 HD | 26" + 17" side | 5 HP gas | 2.6 cu. ft. | 145 lb. |
| American Lincoln A333 | 44" (with side) | 5 HP gas | 5 cu. ft. | 460 lb. |
| American Lincoln A 4410 | 44" | 12.5 HP gas | 12 cu. ft. | 1975 lb. (ride) |
| Somerset ERS 36E | 36" + 11" side | 1½ HP (battery) | 7 cu. ft. | 1385 lb. (ride) |
| Somerset ERS 36 | 36" + 11" side | 7 HP gas | 7 cu. ft. | 985 lb. (ride) |
| American Lincoln A 1436 | 48" (with side) | 9.2 HP gas | 9 cu. ft. | 1350 lb. (ride) |
| American Lincoln A1440 | 48" | 9.2 HP gas | 12 cu. ft. | 1400 lb. (ride) |
| American Lincoln A 4416 | 56" (with side) | 12.5 HP gas | 12 cu. ft. | 2015 lb. (ride) |
| American Lincoln A 4426 | 56" (with side) | 18 HP gas | 12 cu. ft. | 2030 lb. (ride) |
| American Lincoln A 1438 | 60" (with 2 sides) | 9.2 HP gas | 9 cu. ft. | 1400 lb. (ride) |
| American Lincoln A 1446 | 60" (with side) | 9.2 HP gas | 12 cu. ft. | 1450 lb. (ride) |
| Somerset 42 | 26" 2 x 17" side | 1½ HP (battery) | 2½ cu. ft. | 344 lb. without batteries |

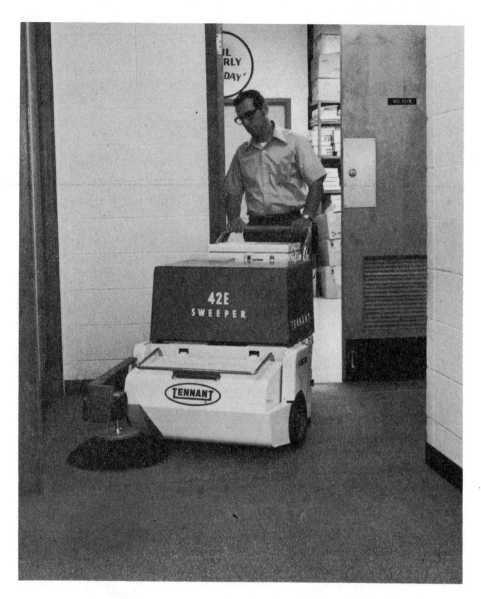

Plate 3
Tennant 42 E Battery Powered Sweeper (Courtesy of Tennant Company, 721 N. Lilac
Drive, Minnneapolis, Minn. 55440)

**Table 5.3 (cont.)**

| Model | Brush width | Power (brush/vacuum) | Capacity | Weight |
|-------|-------------|----------------------|----------|--------|
| Tennant 86 | 42" + 21" side | 18 HP gas | 14 cu. ft. | 1850 lb. (ride) |
| American Lincoln A 4418 | 68" (with 2 sides) | 12.5 HP gas | 12 cu. ft. | 2065 lb. (ride) |
| American Lincoln A 4428 | 68" (with 2 sides) | 18 HP gas | 12 cu. ft. | 2080 lb. (ride) |
| American Lincoln A1448 | 72" (with 2 sides) | 9.2 HP gas | 12 cu. ft. | 1500 lb. (ride) |
| Tennant 92* | 50" + 26" side | 70 HP gas | 23.9 cu. ft. | 4100 lb. (ride) |

main broom, and to sweep material out of gutters, etc., which the machine cannot approach with its main broom. A very large machine can sweep and vacuum 200,000 square feet per hour.

A similar machine that uses carpet beating action instead of sweeping is equipped with a series of straps on a horizontal rotor; these beat the carpet over 20,000 times per minute, and the dust thus shaken out is picked up by a ¾ HP vacuum.

## SCRUBBERS, POLISHERS, AND SCARIFIERS

For many purposes, it is desirable to have a machine that can mechanize the very heavy work of applying friction to a floor finish, whether this is to scrub, polish, or scrape off dirt. While the vacuum sweepers considered in the last section usually have enough power applied to their brushes to do a small amount of buffing or polishing, it is obvious that far greater power is necessary for heavy-duty scrubbing or buffing over large areas. It is also useful to have some means of metering liquids such as detergent solution, liquid polish or other fluids.

In a brushing machine, the disposition of the brushes is a matter of great importance for the efficiency of the process. There are currently three important methods of brush layout that are favored by competing manufacturers, and therefore all three methods tend to have enthusiastic

*See Plate 4.

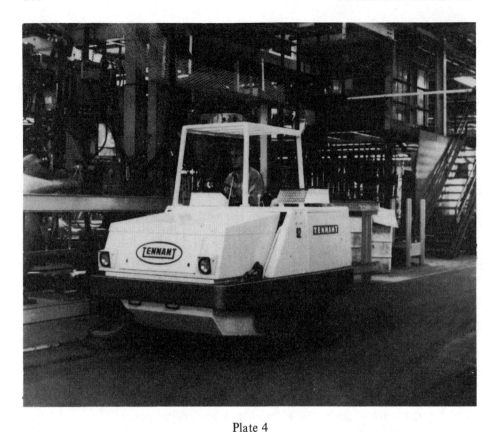

Plate 4
Tennant 92 Sweeper (Courtesy of Tennant Company, 721 N. Lilac Drive, Minneapolis Minn. 55440)

proponents. The methods can be classified as single-brush, two-brush counter-rotating, and three-brush.

### SINGLE-BRUSH MACHINES

In the single-brush machine the motor, through suitable gear or belts, drives a central shaft at the desired speed. A single circular brush is fitted directly to this shaft. The advantages in mechanical efficiency are obvious: the connection is simple, and converts a very large proportion of the motor torque into useful work on the floor. The weight of the motor, gearing, and housing are of necessity directly over the center of the brush, and therefore lend firmness and stability to the brushing action. The disadvantage is that there is a tendency for the motor torque to act also on the body of the machine, swinging it round in the opposite direction to that of the brush, and this torque has to be corrected by the operator holding the handle of the machine; if this were released and the motor went on turning, the handle would swing round and round. For this reason nearly all the machines are fitted with a "dead-man's handle" type of switch that cuts out immediately when pressure is released. Many machines have dual switch levers, usable with either hand, to avoid fatigue. A large machine can be very difficult to manage, but the skilled operator's technique is to allow the torque of the machine to move it from side to side, rather than pushing it or struggling against it.

Machines of this type can be obtained with a wide variety of brush diameters. Table 5.4 lists the most important machines.

**Table 5.4 Scrubbing Machines**

| *Model* | *Brush diameter* | *Brush RPM* | *HP* | *Weight* | *Tank* |
|---|---|---|---|---|---|
| Clarke FM 12 | 12" | 175 | 1/3 | 31 lb. | —— |
| Advance Gyro II | 12" | 195 | 1/3 | 40 lb. | 1 1/2 gal. |
| Hild P 12 | 12" | 185 | 1/3 | 43 lb. | 2 gal. |
| Clarke FM 13 | 13" | 175 | 1/3 | 36 lb. | 2 gal. |
| Clarke S 13 | 13" | 175 | 1/2 | 64 lb. | 4 gal. |
| General Floor-craft KC 12 | 13" | 180 | 1/3 | 56 lb. | 2, 3¼ or 4 gal. |
| General Floor-craft KL 13 | 13" | 180 | 1/3 or 1/2 | 45-49 lb. | 2, 3¼ or 4 gal. |
| General Floor-craft KH 12 | 13" | 180 | 1/4 | 57 lb. | |
| Hild P 13 | 13" | 185 | 1/3 | 48 lb. | 3 gal. |
| Advance Gyro II | 14" | 195 | 1/3 | 45 lb. | 1 1/2 gal. |
| Atlas Fleet-wood FC/-FR 144 | 14" | 175 | 1/2 | 95 lb. | |
| Hild P 14 | 14" | 185 | 1/3 | 54 lb. | 3 gal. |
| Nobles Speed-shine 1433 MD | 14" | 175 | 1/3 | 65 lb. | 3 gal. |
| Nobles Speed-shine 1450 MD | 14" | 175 | 1/2 | 70 lb. | 3 gal. |

**Table 5.4 (cont.)**

| Model | Brush diameter | Brush RPM | HP | Weight | Tank |
|---|---|---|---|---|---|
| Nobles Speed-shine 1450 SD | 14" | 175 | 1/2 | 80 lb. | 3 gal. |
| Nobles Speed-shine 1450 DX | 14" | 175 | 1/2 | 85 lb. | 3 gal. |
| Advance Centurion | 15" | 177 | 3/4 | 87 lb. | |
| Advance Pacemaker II | 15" | 177 | 3/4 | 98 lb. | |
| Atlas CR 155 | 15" | 180 | 3/4 | 90 lb. | |
| Breuer Tornado 15-1 | 15" | 175 | 1 | 92 lb. | |
| Clarke FM 15 | 15" | 175 | 3/4 | 94 lb. | 4 gal. |
| Clarke S 15 | 15" | 175 | 3/4 | 95 lb. | 4 gal. |
| General Floorcraft KC/-KR 14 | 15" | 160 | 1/3 or 1/2 | 82-95 lb. | 2, 3¼ or 4 gal. |
| General Floorcraft KL 15 | 15" | 180 | 1/3 or 1/2 | 48-52 lb. | 2, 3¼ or 4 gal. |
| General Floorcraft GF-15 A and B | 15" | 180 | 1/3 or 1/2 | 66-80 lb. | |
| National SP-15 | 15" | 175 | 1/2 | 95 lb. | 3 gal. |
| World Wildcat 150 | 15" | 177 | 3/4 | 92 lb. | 4 gal. |
| Advance Galaxie II | 16" | 177 | 1/2 | 80 lb. | |
| Atlas Fleetwood FC/-FR 164 | 16" | 175 | 1/2 | 103 lb. | |
| Atlas Fleetwood FC/-FR 165 | 16" | 175 | 3/4 | 107 lb. | |
| Clarke S 16 | 16" | 175 | 3/4 | 98 lb. | 4 gal. |
| Floorola Colt 316 A | 16" | 172 | 1/2 | 80 lb. | 3 1/2 gal. |
| Floorola Colt 316 B | 16" | 172 | 3/4 | 85 lb. | 3 1/2 gal. |

**Table 5.4 (cont.)**

| Model | Brush diameter | Brush RPM | HP | Weight | Tank |
|---|---|---|---|---|---|
| Floorola Stallion 516 A | 16" | 172 | 1/2 | 89 lb. | 3 1/2 gal. |
| Floorola Stallion 516 B | 16" | 172 | 3/4 | 92 lb. | 3 1/2 gal. |
| Floorola Stallion 516 C | 16" | 172 | 1 | 106 lb. | 3 1/2 gal. |
| Floorola One-Pass 816 | 16" | 114 | 1 1/2 | 120 lb. | 3 1/2 gal. |
| Floorola Stallion 503 C | 16", 19" or 22" | 172 | 1 | 102 lb. (with 16" brush) | 3 1/2 gal. |
| Hild P 16 | 16" | 185 | 1/2 | 70 lb. | 3 gal. |
| Hild UP 16 | 16" | 185 | 3/4 | 75 lb. | 3 gal. |
| National Floortainer | 16" | 175 | 1/2 | 78 lb. | 3 gal. |
| Advance Centurion | 17" | 177 | 1 | 95 lb. | |
| Advance Pacemaker II | 17" | 177 | 1 | 106 lb. | |
| Atlas FC/FR 175 | 17" | 175 | 3/4 | 110 lb. | |
| Atlas CR 175 | 17" | 180 | 3/4 | 95 lb. | |
| Breuer Tornado 17-1 | 17" | 175 | 1 | 95 lb. | |
| Clarke FM 17 | 17" | 175 | 3/4 | 96 lb. | 4 gal. |
| General Floorcraft KC/-KR 16 | 17" | 160 | 1/2 or 3/4 | 86-106 lb. | 2, 3¼ or 4 gal. |
| General Floorcraft GF-17 A and B | 17" | 180 | 1/2 or 3/4 | 71-90 lb. | 2, 3¼ or 4 gal. |
| National SP-17 | 17" | 175 | 3/4 | 100 lb. | 3 gal. |
| Nobles Speedshine 1775 MD | 17" | 175 | 3/4 | 85 lb. | 3 gal. |
| Nobles Speedshine 1775 SD | 17" | 175 | 3/4 | 90 lb. | 3 gal. |

**Table 5.4 (cont.)**

| Model | Brush diameter | Brush RPM | HP | Weight | Tank |
|---|---|---|---|---|---|
| Nobles Speed-shine 1775 DX | 17" | 175 | 3/4 | 95 lb. | 3 gal. |
| World Wildcat 170 | 17" | 177 | 1 | 102 lb. | 4 gal. |
| Advance Galaxie II | 18" | 177 | 3/4 | 86 lb. | |
| Clarke S 18 | 18" | 175 | 1 | 105 lb. | 4 gal. |
| Hild P 18 | 18" | 185 | 3/4 | 80 lb. | 3 gal. |
| Atlas Fleet-wood FC/-FR 195 | 19" | 175 | 3/4 | 112 lb. | |
| Atlas Fleet-wood FC/FR 196 | 19" | 175 | 1 | 120 lb. | |
| Atlas Fleet-wood CR 195 | 19" | 180 | 3/4 | 100 lb. | |
| Atlas Fleet-wood CR 196 | 19" | 180 | 1 | 104 lb. | |
| Breuer Tor-nado 19-1 1/3 | 19" | 173 | 1 1/3 | 103 lb. | |
| Floorola Colt 319B | 19" | 172 | 3/4 | 90 lb. | 3 1/2 gal. |
| Floorola Stal-lion 519 B | 19" | 172 | 3/4 | 96 lb. | 3 1/2 gal. |
| Floorola Stal-lion 519 C | 19" | 172 | 1 | 112 lb. | 3 1/2 gal. |
| Floorola One-Pass | 19" | 114 | 1 1/2 | 130 lb. | 3 1/2 gal. |
| General Floor-craft KC/-KR 18 | 19" | 160 | 3/4 or 1 | 99-121 lb. | 2, 3¼ or 4 gal. |
| General Floor-craft GF-19A | 19" | 180 | 3/4 or 1 | 88-93 lb. | |

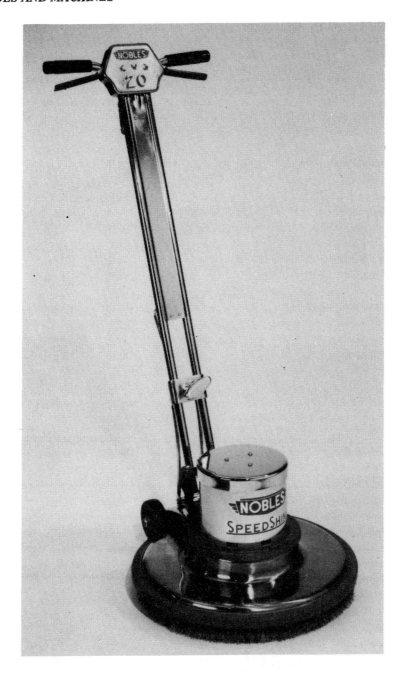

Plate 5
Nobles 20" Three Star Speedshine Floor Polishing and Scrubbing Machine (Courtesy
of Nobles Industries Incorporated, 645 East 7th Street, St. Paul, Minn. 55106)

**Table 5.4 (cont.)**

| Model | Brush diameter | Brush RPM | HP | Weight | Tank |
|-------|----------------|-----------|-----|--------|------|
| National Floor-tainer | 19" | 175 | 3/4 | 88 lb. | 3 gal. |
| Advance Centurion | 20" | 177 | 1 1/4 | 111 lb. | |
| Advance Pacemaker II | 20" | 177 | 1 1/4 | 122 lb. | |
| Advance Galaxie II | 20" | 177 | 1 | 93 lb. | |
| Clarke FM 20 | 20" | 175 | 1 | 110 lb. | 4 gal. |
| Clarke S 20 | 20" | 175 | 1 | 166 lb. | 4 gal. |
| National SP-20 | 20" | 175 | 1 | 114 lb. | 3 gal. |
| Nobles Speed-shine 2075 MD | 20" | 175 | 3/4 | 90 lb. | 3 gal. |
| Nobles Speed-shine 2075 SD | 20" | 175 | 3/4 | 100 lb. | 3 gal. |
| Nobles Speed-shine 2001 SD | 20" | 175 | 1 | 105 lb. | 3 gal. |
| Nobles Speed-shine 2075 DX | 20" | 175 | 3/4 | 105 lb. | 3 gal. |
| Nobles Speed-shine 2001 DX | 20" | 175 | 1 | 110 lb. | 3 gal. |
| Nobles Three-Star Speed-shine * 20001-3 | 20" | 175 | 1 | 120 lb. | 3 1/2 gal. |
| World Wildcat 200 | 20" | 177 | 1 1/4 | 114 lb. | 4 gal. |
| General Floorcraft KC/-KR 20 | 21" | 160 | 3/4 or 1 | 106-123 lb. | 2, 3¼ or 4 gal. |
| General Floorcraft GF-21A | 21" | 160 | 3/4 or 1 | 101-108 lb. | 2, 3¼ or 4 gal. |

*See Plate 5.

**Table 5.4 (cont.)**

| Model | Brush diameter | Brush RPM | HP | Weight | Tank |
|---|---|---|---|---|---|
| Advance Pace-maker II | 22" | 177 | 1 1/4 | 122 lb. | |
| Atlas Fleet-wood FC/-FR 226 | 22" | 165 | 1 | 130 lb. | |
| Atlas Fleet-wood CR 226 | 22" | 180 | 1 | 108 lb. | |
| Breuer Tor-nado 22-1 1/3 | 22" | 173 | 1 1/3 | 107 lb. | |
| Floorola Stal-lion 522 C | 22" | 154 | 1 | 124 lb. | 3 1/2 gal. |
| World Wild-cat 220 | 22" | 177 | 1 1/4 | 106 lb. | 4 gal. |
| Clarke FM 23 | 23" | 175 | 1 | 137 lb. | 4 gal. |
| General Floor-craft KC/-KR 22 | 23" | 160 | 1 | 111-130 lb. | 2, 3¼ or 4 gal. |
| General Floor-craft GF-23A | 23" | 160 | 1 | 110 lb. | 2, 3¼ or 4 gal. |
| Nobles Speed-shine 2301 SD | 23" | 175 | 1 | 115 lb. | 3 gal. |
| Nobles Speed-shine 2301 DX | 23" | 175 | 1 | 120 lb. | 3 gal. |

The capacity of such a machine, in terms of scrubbing or polishing a given area of floor, is obviously affected by the degree of congestion, furniture, sharp bends, and so on, that obstruct an easy flow of work. However, in general, over a clear working area the user can expect to *polish* about 3800 square feet per hour for every square foot of brush surface. Thus a 13-inch diameter brush (actual working area around 126 square inches or 0.87 square feet) will polish up to 3300 square feet per hour, a 15-inch brush up to 4750 square feet, a 17-inch brush up to 6000 square feet, and a 22-inch brush up to 10,000 square feet. The fact that the work done increases with the square of the brush diameter makes it even more important to choose the largest machine that can reasonably be "navigated" on any particular premises. This is, in fact, the cardinal rule for selection of all machines in the cleaning field.

Scrubbing will not usually be such a rapid job as polishing, but the same principle applies. The buyer, in judging a demonstration of a scrubbing machine, should take particular note of the means for applying detergent solution. The tank should be large enough to hold all the liquid needed for the largest single area in the premises, and the position of the liquid supply to the brushes should be such as to minimize splashing from the edges of the brushes. Most of the machines above have feed arrangements to the center of the brush, or through a perforated brush. The liquid feed must have positive control of flow, particularly important for carpet shampooing and the treatment of surfaces sensitive to moisture, such as cork.

All brushing machines should have means for raising the brushes from the floor; most single-brush machines tilt backwards. When the machine is put away, it should always be stored with the brushes up to minimize crushing of the brush bristles.

## TWO-BRUSH MACHINES

The great disadvantage of the single-brush machine is the uneven torque distribution, so that the machine tends to turn counter to the brush rotation. In a large machine this may be a considerable force, and women should not be expected to control, say, a 22-inch single-brush machine. Furthermore, single-brush machines of the larger type may be a hazard in premises where there is delicate equipment or furniture, because even with a powerful operator they can still run away a little.

The obvious solution to this difficulty is to have two brushes rotating counter to one another so that the torque is equalized. Given equal wear on the bristles and a smooth surface, there is no reason why a machine of this design should not run smoothly even without an operator. While this may not be achieved in practice, the two-brush machine is very easy to control.

The main *disadvantages* of the two-brush machine are:

1. The drive from a motor shaft to two brushes is necessarily more complicated than the direct drive to one brush. If friction is used to drive the second brush, there is danger of slipping and loss of power. If gears are used, the machine becomes more expensive and the gears themselves consume power.

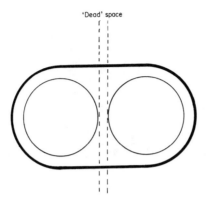

Figure 5.2

Two-brush cleaning mechanism, showing the "dead" space between the two brushes.

2. The second disadvantage is that the line down the middle of the machine, passing through the point where the brushes are closest together, is hardly scrubbed or polished at all, except by the very edges of the brushes, and therefore far more overlapping of machine paths is necessary than with the single-brush machine (see Figure 5.2).

You may purchase two-brush machines that are specially recommended for "delicate" areas and for use by women. Typical examples are a ½ HP model with a total 21-inch brush spread, weighing 86 pounds and a ½ HP model with 16-inch brush spread, weighing 31 pounds. These machines are eminently suitable for smaller premises, such as stores and hairdressers' salons, and for premises with fragile goods or apparatus, such as laboratories.

Large two-brush machines are not much in demand, as the "dead space" between the brushes tends to counteract any advantages of the greater width.

### THREE-BRUSH MACHINES

The simplest way to obviate the gap in the two-brush models is to add another brush along the center line. This reintroduces the problems of uneven torque, and adds to the problems of drive; friction drive becomes even more inefficient if applied to three brushes, and geared drives are more expensive. Figure 5.3, however, shows a very ingenious adaptation of the three-brush design called the "torqueless three-brush system"; it combines the qualities of the conventional three-brush layout with some of the advantages of the single-brush layout.

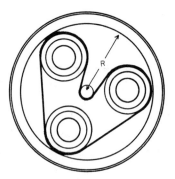

Figure 5.3

Three-brush system, Cimex Ltd. A belt passes around the central driving shaft and the three brushes, which are mounted on a circular plate which is free to revolve.

Three brushes are arranged at the corners of an equilateral triangle on a circular plate. The brushes are free to revolve on their own axes, and the plate is also free to revolve independently of the main drive shaft. A belt passes around this drive shaft and the three brushes. The action of the torqueless system is best understood by considering the extreme cases of its action. If the load on the brushes is infinitely small, so that they are completely free to revolve, they will take up the full movement of the belt and the plate will not revolve at all. In fact, the machine will behave like a conventional three-brush machine with the brushes fixed in a triangular layout. The speed of the brushes will be in simple ratio of the radius of the brush to the radius of the drive shaft.

If, at the other end of the scale, the load on the brushes is so great that they cannot rotate at all around their own centers, all the pull of the belt will tend to make the circular table revolve, and the machine will then behave like a single-brush machine with one large brush of radius R (which just happens to be interrupted at intervals). The speed of rotation will be the ratio of R to the radius of the drive shaft, and therefore less than half the speed of rotation of the brushes in the first case considered. In practice, the motion of the machine is always a combination of the two movements, but if the load is light, as in polishing, most of the belt drive will go into rapid rotations of the brushes with slow rotations of the plate. If the load is heavy, as in scrubbing or removing grease or mud, the torque will go into slower rotations of the table, and the brushes will not turn very rapidly. The machine in this latter case behaves like a slow-speed single-brush model. This variation in speed is very useful, as polishing needs a fairly light, rapid movement, while scrubbing needs a slower speed and more force. The torqueless system thus behaves as if it were an automatic, infinitely variable gear.

Figure 5.4 illustrates details of the mechanism; Plate 6 shows the Cimex range of machines using this system. The four machines have the specifications set out in Table 5.5.

**Table 5.5 Specifications of Cimex Three-Brush Machines**

|  | *R76* | *R61* | *R48* | *R38* |
|---|---|---|---|---|
| Working diameter | 30" | 24" | 19" | 15" |
| Weight | 185½ lb. | 147 lb. | 106½ lb. | 76½ lb. |
| HP | 1½ | 1 | 2/3 | ½ |
| Average area/- hr (polishing) | 20,000 ft.$^2$ | 12,000 ft.$^2$ | 6000 ft.$^2$ | 4000 ft.$^2$ |

It will be found that the coverage per hour, as specified by the manufacturers, follows the approximate rule stated earlier (3800 square feet per hour for every square foot of brush area) if the torqueless system is assumed to behave like a single-brush system of the same overall diameter.

## Scarifying

The removal of heavy grease, often packed with sawdust and metal chips, mud, and other thick deposits from floors, is a matter of concern to many branches of the food trade, engineering and building concerns, and paint-spray shops. Most ordinary scrubbers fail in this work because the brushes soon become clogged with sticky deposits and just skim over the surface, and many machines are not powerful enough to keep the bristles moving if they do bite into the soil. On the other hand, the deposits obviously cannot be left too long; they are a serious hazard to health and safety. Blood-soaked sawdust, for example, in a slaughter house or butchershop may be the ideal breeding ground for bacteria of all kinds, flies, and other insects. Grease, paint, and plastic spills (epoxy resin, for example) can cause expensive and avoidable industrial accidents.

Suppliers of the heavier type of floor machine can supply special wire brushes for scarifying. To avoid clogging with grease and similar matter, the bristles are set wider apart than in the conventional brush, and have spaces to allow the collected soil to fall out of the brush. These are not suitable for the lighter type of machine, and in any case the machine should have a motor in the 3/4-1 HP range to cope with the heavy loading on such a heavy-duty scrubber.

An alternative method of scarifying simulates the scraping action of a

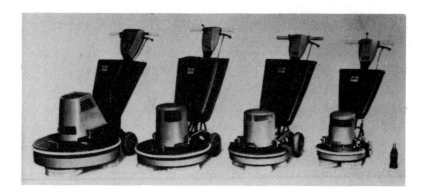

Plate 6
R 76, R 61, R 48, R 38 Floor Machines (Courtesy of Cimex International, Orpington, Kent BR5 3PX England)

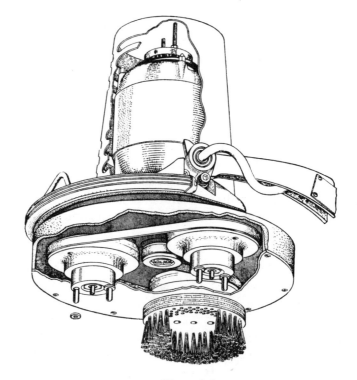

Figure 5.4

Cimex torqueless three-brush system. (Acknowledgments to Cimex Ltd.)

chisel or trowel. The four blades are driven with reciprocating motion by a ½ HP engine (gas or electric) over a 15-inch path width. The blades have slight "float" and some freedom to move right or left, to allow the machine to follow slight irregularities in the floor surface and to run along tile edges. The weight is 154 pounds (electric), 160 pounds (gas). It should be followed by an efficient large vacuum cleaner or sweeper to pick up the scraping.

For really large areas, the automatic machines considered later are all adapted to use scarifying brushes and pick up the debris themselves.

## SUCTION DRYERS

One of the greatest difficulties in the cleaning of premises, compared with that of, say, articles of clothing or tableware, is that rinsing and drying are difficult to carry out, and tend to be the most inefficient part of the operation. Mechanical scrubbers may take the manual labor out of the application of detergent, but too often the dirty cleaning solution is left on the floor to dry out slowly and streakily. The suction dryer is the answer to this problem.

The idea of a vacuum cleaner that will pick up water as well as dust is obviously a good one; the difficulties come in designing a fan system that will give adequate suction for water without the water coming into contact with the motor or other electrical parts. Manufacturers have solved this problem by making "by-pass" motors, so that machines are now available to pick up wet and dry debris without either coming into the motor housing.

For efficient wet pick-up the usual fitting is a narrow nozzle with a squeegee blade to assist in drying. Some large machines are available which fit over a 55-gallon drum, for use in clearing flooded areas or salvaging spilled material. Table 5.6 gives details of some of the large range of suction dryers on the U.S. market.

**Table 5.6 Suction Dryers**

| Model | Wet capacity | HP | Water-lift | CFM | Weight |
|---|---|---|---|---|---|
| Breuer Tornado PRO | ½ gal. | 1.1 | 37" | 69 | 16½ lb. |
| Clarke 600A General Floorcraft | 2½ gal. | 1 | 63" | | 26 lb. |
| Minivac G-2 Breuer Tornado | 3 gal. | 1 | 55" | 100 | 18 lb. |
| 140/1 | 3 gal. | 1.1 | 39" | 80 | 24½ lb. |

**Table 5.6 (cont.)**

| Model | Wet capacity | HP | Water-lift | CFM | Weight |
|---|---|---|---|---|---|
| National Colt | 3 gal. | 1 | 47" | 168 | 29 lb. |
| Advance Pacesetter J-105 | 5 gal. | ¾ | | | 39 lb. |
| Advance Pacesetter SJ-105 | 5 gal. | ¾ | | | 46 lb. |
| Breuer Tornado 144/5 | 5 gal. | 1.1 | 39" | 80 | 25 lb. |
| World Warrior 50 | 5 gal. | ¾ | 80" | | 43 lb. |
| Hild 404 | 6 gal. | | 90" | 89 | 19½ lb. |
| Hild 604 | 6 gal. | | 96" | 94 | 19½ lb. |
| Nobles 680 | 6 gal. | ½ | | | 41 lb. |
| General Floor-craft G-10A | 7 gal. | 1 | 79" | 80 | 29 lb. |
| National Colt | 7 gal. | 1 | 47" | 168 | 37 lb. |
| Advance Pacesetter J-108 | 8 gal. | ¾ | | | 41 lb. |
| Advance Pacesetter SJ-108 | 8 gal. | ¾ | | | 48 lb. |
| World Warrior 80 | 8 gal. | ¾ | 80" | | 45 lb. |
| Clarke 609 | 9 gal. | 1 | 65" | | 44½ lb. |
| Breuer Tornado 310/320 | 10 gal. | 1¾ | 44" | 111 | 68 lb. |
| Breuer Tornado 250 | 10 gal. | 1¾ | 50" | 103 | 52½ lb. |
| Breuer Tornado 410/440 | 10 gal. | 7/8 | 30" | 111 | 45-57 lb. |
| Breuer Tornado 420/450 | 10 gal. | 1½ | 37" | 118 | 49-61 lb. |
| Breuer Tornado 430/460 | 10 gal. | 2 | 47" | 144 | 51-63 lb. |
| Hild 706-1½ | 10 gal. | 1½ | 68" | 250 | 50 lb. |
| Hild 406 | 10 gal. | | 90" | 89 | 33 lb. |
| Hild 606 | 10 gal | | 96" | 94 | 33 lb. |
| Nobles Speedry V24B | 10 gal. | ¾ | | 76 | 82 lb. |
| Atlas Vac-Mop | 10-15 gal. | 1½ | 78" | | 82-91 lb. |
| Atlas Vac-/Cleen | 10-15 gal. | 1½ | 78-80" | | 90-103 lb. |
| Advance Hydrovac 112/212 | 12 gal. | 1 | 78" | | 57 lb. |
| Advance Hydrovac SL112/212 | 12 gal | 1 | 78" | | 71 lb. |

**Table 5.6 (cont.)**

| Model | Wet capacity | HP | Water-lift | CFM | Weight |
|---|---|---|---|---|---|
| Advance Pacesetter J-1200 | 12 gal. | ¾ | | | 53 lb. |
| Advance Pacesetter SLJ-1200 | 12 gal. | ¾ | | | 66 lb. |
| Advance Triumph TR-112 | 12 gal. | 1 1/3 | | | 59 lb. |
| Advance Triumph SLTR-112 | 12 gal. | 1 1/3 | | | 73 lb. |
| General Floorcraft 57 | 12 gal. | 1½ | 92" | | 70 lb. |
| World Warrior 120 | 12 gal. | 1¼ | 98" | | 62 lb. |
| Nobles 1200T | 12 gal. | 1½ | 100" | | 54-62 lb. |
| Clarke 612 | 12 gal. | 1½ | 100" | | 68 lb. |
| Nobles Wet-n-Dry | 12½ gal. | | | 89.6 | 53 lb. |
| National Colt | 12½ gal. | 1 | 47" | 168 | 36-46 lb. |
| Hild 715-1½ | 15 gal. | 1½ | 68" | 250 | 64 lb. |
| Hild 415 | 15 gal. | | 90" | 89 | 43 lb. |
| Hild 615 | 15 gal. | | 96" | 94 | 43 lb. |
| General Floorcraft 77 | 15 gal. | 1 | 79" | 137 | 59 lb. |
| General Floorcraft 99 | 15 gal. | 1½ | 92" | 170 | 62 lb. |
| National Super SH | 15 gal. | 1¼ | 30" | 243 | 49 lb. |
| Advance SL116/-216 | 16 gal. | 1 | 78" | | 73 lb. |
| Advance Pacesetter J-1600 | 16 gal. | ¾ | | | 56 lb. |
| Advance Pacesetter SLJ-1600 | 16 gal. | ¾ | | | 69 lb. |
| Advance Triumph TR-116 | 16 gal. | 1 1/3 | | | 62 lb. |
| Advance Triumph SLTR 116 | 16 gal | 1 1/3 | | | 76 lb. |
| World Warrior 160 | 16 gal. | 1¼ | 98" | | 67 lb. |
| National Hustler | 19 gal. | 1½ | 45" | 212 | 53-65 lb. |
| Hild 730-1½ | 30 gal. | 1½ | 68" | 250 | 79 lb. |
| Hild 430 | 30 gal. | | 90" | 89 | 72 lb. |
| Hild 630 | 30 gal. | | 96" | 94 | 72 lb. |
| Hild 755-1½ | 55 gal. | 1½ | 68" | 250 | 88 lb. |
| Hild 765-1½ | 55 gal. | 2 x 1½ | 68" | 500 | 117 lb. |
| Hild 655 | 55 gal. | | 96" | 94 | |

**Table 5.6 (cont.)**

| Model | Wet capacity | HP | Water-lift | CFM | Weight |
|-------|--------------|-----|-----------|-----|--------|
| Advance Triumph TR 102X | 55 gal. | 1 1/3 | | | 38 lb. without drum |
| Advance Triumph TR 103X | 55 gal. | 1 1/3 | | | 60 lb. without drum |

Most of these machines are also suitable for dry suction, and can thus be classed as general-purpose vacuum cleaners. Such a machine may be the answer to the cleaning problems of many premises, although it must be remembered that the by-pass motor and other features tend to make wet-suction machines heavier than dry vacuum cleaners of similar power and capacity. Where the machine has to be taken up stairs, this may be a disadvantage. The large machines, especially those adapted to fit over a standard 55-gallon drum, are suitable for such jobs as boiler-tube cleaning, clearing the cutting oils out of the sumps of lathes, and similar work. If the residues are at all noxious, the drums can be sealed and discarded when full, while the machine itself can be decontaminated by running warm detergent solution through it.

## AUTOSCRUBBERS

For the really large plant, the ideal machine is one that scrubs, polishes if necessary, and dries the floor, all in one pass, using one operator. Such machines may be called collectively *autoscrubbers*, and several models are available with varying capacities over a wide range of floor area. The conventional design is a machine with a brush or brushes at the front for scrubbing, and a wet-suction squeegee system at the rear which picks up the dirty water and leaves the floor dry. The machines may also be used to clean and burnish with emulsion polish.

Table 5.7 summarizes the main models on the market.

## CHOICE OF MACHINES

With so many different types of machines on the market and so many excellent models within each class, the maintenance manager who has to make a buying decision (whether to replace existing machines, to

**Table 5.7 Autoscrubbers**

| *Model* | *Total brush width* | *Sq. Ft./hr.* | *Solution tank capacity* | *Recovery tank capacity* | *Vacuum motor HP* | *Brush motor HP* | *Weight* | *Squeegee width* | *Brush pressure* | *Length* |
|---|---|---|---|---|---|---|---|---|---|---|
| Breuer Tornado 3500 | 16" | | 8.6 gal. | 10.6 gal. | ¾ | ½ | 590 lb. | 21" | 30-80 lb. | 47" battery |
| Clarke Mini-Matic | 16" | 6,000 | 3½ gal. | 4 gal. | 1 | | 95 lb. | 19½" | | 27" mains |
| Advance Convert-amatic 17E | 17" | 13,000 | 11 gal. | 10 gal. | ¾ | ½ | 198 lb. | 20½" | 65 lb. | 37" mains |
| Advance Convert-amatic 18B II | 18" | 13,000 | 10 gal. | 8 gal. | ¾ | ½ | 422 lb. | 22" | 70 lb. | 49¼" battery |
| Clarke Compact TB 18 | 18¼" | 14,000 | 10 gal. | 12 gal. | ¾ | ¾ | 595 lb. | 23¼" | 20-80 lb. | 51" battery |
| American-Lincoln Autoscrubber 719-2B | 19" | 12,000 | 10 gal. | 12 gal. | 1/3 | ¾ | 382 lb. | 23" | 30-90 lb. | 45" battery |
| Advance Convert-amatic 20E | 20" | 15,500 | 11 gal. | 10 gal. | ¾ | ¾ | 232 lb. | 22" | 70 lb. | 38¾" mains |
| Clarke Compact PE-20 | 20" | 10,000 | 9 gal. | 12 gal. | 1 | ¾ | 255 lb. | 23½" | 80 lb. | 39¼" mains |
| Clarke Compact PS-20 BP | 20" | 15,480 | 10 gal. | 12 gal. | | ¾ | 675 lb. | 23½" | 48-94 lb. | 51½" battery |
| World Whirl-amatic 200E | 20" | 15,000 | 9 gal. | 8 gal. | ¾ | ¾ | 232 lb. | 22" | | mains |
| Advance Convert-amatic 21B | 21" | 15,500 | 10 gal. | 8 gal. | ¾ | 0.8 | 494 lb. | 26" | 90-130 lb. | 50" battery |
| American-Lincoln Autoscrubber 621 CE | 21" | 15,000 | 8½ gal. | 12 gal. | | 1¼ | 234 lb. | 23" | 70-120 lb. | 38½" mains |

**Table 5.7 (cont.)**

| Model | Total brush width | Sq. Ft./hr. | Solution tank capacity | Recovery tank capacity | Vacuum Motor HP | Brush motor HP | Weight | Squeegee width | Brush pressure | Length |
|---|---|---|---|---|---|---|---|---|---|---|
| American-Lincoln Autoscrubber 721-2B | 21" | 15,000 | 16 gal. | 16 gal. | 1/3 | 0.8 | 920 lb. | 23" | 115 lb. | 54" battery |
| Hild Double-Duty Scrubber-Vac | 21" | 17,000 | 12 gal. | 12 gal. | 1 | | 725 lb. | 26" | 48-68 lb. | 51" battery |
| World Whirl-amatic 210B | 21" | 15,500 | 10 gal. | 8 gal. | 3/4 | 0.8 | 528 lb. | 26" | 90-130 lb. | 42" battery |
| Advance Convert-amatic 24E | 24" | 17,000 | 15 gal. | 15 gal. | 3/4 | 3/4 | 445 lb. | 28" | 100-130 lb. | 42" mains |
| Advance Convert-amatic 24B | 24" | 17,000 | 15 gal. | 15 gal. | 3/4 | 0.8 | 666 lb. | 28" | 120-200 lb. | 50" battery |
| Breuer Tornado 3800 | 24" | | 15 gal. | 17 gal. | 3/4 | 0.8 | 880 lb. | 29" | 75-145 lb. | 56⅛" battery |
| World Whirl-amatic 240B | 24" | 17,000 | 15 gal. | 15 gal. | 3/4 | 0.8 | 650 lb. | 28" | 120-200 lb. | 42" battery |
| World Whirl-amatic 240E | 24" | 17,000 | 15 gal. | 15 gal. | 3/4 | 3/4 | 445 lb. | 28" | | mains |
| Clarke TB 24 | 24½" | 22,500 | 15 gal. | 20 gal. | 3/4 | 2x½ | 1140 lb. | 30" | 60-100 lb. | 60" battery |
| American-Lincoln Autoscrubber 726-2B | 26" | 18,000 | 16 gal. | 16 gal. | 1/3 | 1.3 | 950 lb. | 31" | 140 lb. | 52½" battery |
| American-Lincoln Autoscrubber 730-2B | 30" | 25,000 | 16 gal. | 16 gal. | 1/3 | 1.3 | 980 lb. | 35" | 130 lb. | 55" battery |

126

**Table 5.7 (cont.)**

| Model | Total brush width | Sq. Ft./hr. | Solution tank capacity | Recovery tank capacity | Vacuum motor HP | Brush motor HP | Weight | Squeegee width | Brush pressure | Length |
|---|---|---|---|---|---|---|---|---|---|---|
| Advance Convert-amatic 32B | 32" | 25,000 | 24 gal. | 2x12 gal. | 2x¾ | 1.3 | 944 lb. | 36" | 150-225 lb. | 50½" battery |
| World Whirl-amatic 320 BD | 32" | 25,000 | 24 gal. | 24 gal. | 2x¾ | 1.3 | 980 lb. | 36" | 150-250 lb. | 48" battery |
| World Whirl-amatic 320 GD | 32" | 25,000 | 24 gal. | 24 gal. | 6 HP | | 660 lb. | 36" | | 48" gasoline |
| Clarke TB 32A | 32½" | 30,000 | 20 gal. | 24 gal. | ¾ | 1½ | 1310 lb. | 36" | 80-200 lb. | 63½" battery |
| Advance Convert-amatic 450B | 45" | 35,000 | 25 gal. | 24 gal. | 2x¾ | 2 | 1590 lb. | 49" | | 64" battery |
| Advance Convert-amatic 450 G | 45" | 35,000 | 32 gal. | 32 gal. | 7 HP | | 1030 lb. | 49" | | 64" gasoline |
| American-Lincoln Scrubmobile 530G | 30" | 27,000 | 18 gal. | 16 gal. | 7 HP | | 760 lb. | 31" | 200 lb. | 56" gasoline |
| American-Lincoln Scrubmobile 538G | 38" | 33,000 | 28 gal. | 25 gal. | 7 HP | | 942 lb. | 38" | 200 lb. | 56" gasoline |
| American-Lincoln Scrubmobile 560G | 60" | 75,000 | 100 gal. | 80 gal. | 14 HP | | 2350 lb. | 60" | 500 lb. | 115" gasoline |
| American-Lincoln Scrubmobile | 72" | 100,000 | 200 gal. | 210 gal. | 30 HP | | 5800 lb. | 72" | 600 lb. | 136" gasoline |

Weights of battery models are given as with batteries loaded. The American-Lincoln Scrubmobile models are "ride" models: they are also available to run from low-pressure propane gas, and these models are all 50 lb heavier than the corresponding gasoline models.

reorganize the maintenance of a building, or to fit out a new plant altogether) may feel excused for feeling bewildered. The circumstances of every building are different in terms of the type of dirt to be expected, nature of flooring materials, degree of congestion, type of labor available, and minimum standards of hygiene necessary, but a few general hints may act as guidelines in the choice of machines.

1. In general, the aim should be to eliminate hand labor as far as possible and make the greatest use of machines. The machines, however, must not be too unwieldy to handle in the building under normal work conditions, and the maintenance and setting-up of the machines themselves should not take longer than doing the job by hand. This last point is an ever-present danger: management may acquire a new toy in the shape of an expensive piece of equipment, only to find in a month or two that it is being left in its closet or bay, unused, because the brushes take too long to fit, or the machine is difficult to start, or it cannot maneuver through the space between machines or through doorways.

2. Cleaning personnel should be consulted in the *choice* stages; ideally, some responsible person who actually does some of the cleaning should be present when manufacturers' demonstrations are arranged. While the maintenance manager will obviously know best about square feet per hour, working capacity, and other technical matters, the cleaners will know by experience about such tricky matters as the clearance between articles of furniture and the floor, widths of doorways, and position of electrical outlets, and can often help to prevent the purchase of a costly white elephant. It is not really good enough to consult the personnel *after* a machine has been selected.

3. In extensively carpeted buildings, such as offices and hotels, the most useful machine is undoubtedly the vacuum sweeper. The largest machine which can comfortably be used in the building should always be selected, remembering that the productivity of vacuum sweepers, like that of scrubbers, is proportional to the working area of the brushes, or the square of the width or diameter, so that a 20-inch sweeper will cover four times the ground of a 10-inch sweeper in the same time.

4. On cork and linoleum, thermoplastic and PVC tiles, and other surfaces which are best cleaned regularly by application of thin coats of emulsion polish, an efficient scrubber/polisher or floor machine with a controlled liquid feed is the machine to choose. Again, the largest machine possible for the circumstances of the building should be selected, even if this involves a certain amount of hand labor in corners and congested areas.

5. For factory floors, kithcens, and all hard plastic surfaces such as epoxy resin, polyurethane resin, polyester resin and plastic-finished concrete, the ideal combination is a good floor machine and a wet suction cleaner. Most of the day-to-day maintenance can be carried out by application of thin coats of emulsion polish, using the technique of wet-buffing to clean and polish at the same time, and periodic scrubbing can be made a rapid and efficient job by

drying the floor with suction immediately after the scrubber has passed over it. In this way the floor is ready for use in the minimum time, and work is interrupted for only a short time, if at all.

6. In dirty industries, where the floor is constantly covered with dirt such as grease, rubber, and sawdust, a scarifier is an investment that will pay for itself in a very short time. If the premises are small, scarifying brushes can be bought for the floor machine, as long as the machine is fairly powerful and heavy; for greater speed and efficiency, the "chisel action" scarifier is recommended.

7. For restaurants with carpeted floors a vacuum sweeper should be used, but if the floor is uncarpeted, a wet-suction cleaner is very useful, even if congestion from chairs and tables does not permit the use of a mechanical scrubber. Hand mopping, followed by the wet-suction machine, can make a floor clean and hygienic even in the short time between servings.

8. In large areas, where an autoscrubber is the only effective answer to the cleaning problem, the following figures may assist in the selection of the correct size of machine: for areas up to 10,000 square feet, a 19-inch machine is satisfactory; for 10,000-20,000 square feet a 21-inch machine; for 20,000-50,000 square feet a 24-26-inch machine; for 50,000-100,000 square feet a 30-35-inch machine; for 100,000-200,000 square feet a 60-inch machine, and for anything over this scale the largest machine available, which at present means a 72-inch machine.

9. Where the problem is large spaces covered with litter, as in stadiums, parks, and other areas used by the public, especially as spectators, a large battery- or gasoline-driven vacuum cleaner is the only satisfactory solution.

10. If proper use is made of vacuum sweepers and wet-suction machines, the odd jobs can be carried out very easily with a small portable vacuum cleaner. Equipping cleaning personnel with vacuum cleaners that are really easy to carry will encourage them to clean the "awkward areas" that cannot be reached with the large machines.

11. All the equipment should, of course, meet high standards of electrical insulation and safety. When selecting equipment driven by electricity from a power cord, the user should try to obtain foolproof means of winding up the cord, preferably some kind of automatic winder, especially in the case of heavy floor machines and wet-suction equipment, where the consequences of running over the cord could be serious.

12. Machines should be stored in such a way that the brushes and similar parts are allowed to recover from the effects of weight and friction. Scrubbers and vacuum sweepers should be stored with their brushes raised. Spare brushes should be kept flat with their bristles upwards, not resting on their bristles or pressed together in pairs. Wet-suction machines should have their tanks emptied after every use, and the squeegee and fishtail should be wiped over daily with a damp cloth. All tanks and pipework in wet-suction machines and autoscrubbers should be cleaned out weekly with a solution of neutral detergent in hot water.

When polishers have been used with emulsion polish in the tank or reservoir, wash it out immediately with a neutral detergent (preferably a nonionic detergent in hot water, at about ¼ ounce per gallon). Provision for this cleaning and maintenance of machines should form part of the planning for any mechanization of maintenance work. It will add greatly to the trouble-free life of the machines and ensure that the results obtained are always up to standard.

## COSTS

Most maintenance people will agree that mechanical cleaning is cheaper than manual cleaning, except in the very smallest premises, but detailed costs are not always obtainable. Figures produced by the machine manufacturers tend to be optimistic (although quite honestly prepared) because they leave out details of hand work that still needs to be done when the machines are installed. Figures produced by manufacturers of cleaning products tend to belittle the contribution of machines, and may be rather pessimistic from this viewpoint.

Table 5.8 summarizes the relative costs of

1. Manual cleaning
2. Cleaning with a floor machine followed by a suction dryer
3. Cleaning with an autoscrubber

over the same area of floor in a large store, with terrazzo flooring and generous aisles. This, of course, tends to favor machine operation. These

**Table 5.8 Relative Costs of Manual and Mechanical Floor Cleaning**

|  | *Manual* | *Scrubber + suction dryer* | *Autoscrubber* |
|---|---|---|---|
| Area (square feet) | 12,000 | 12,000 | 12,000 |
| Labor force | 5 | 3 | 2 |
| Hours | 3 | 4 | 3 |
| Labor cost (at $2 per hour) | $30.00 | $24.00 | $12.00 |
| Lighting and power | $ 3.00 | $ 4.00 | $ 4.00 |
| Equipment amortization | $ 0.10 | $ 0.50 | $ 1.40 |
| Detergent cost | $ 2.00 | $ 1.50 | $ 1.25 |
| Total daily cost | $35.10 | $30.00 | $18.65 |
| Total cost per annum (261 working days) | $9,161.10 | $7,830.00 | $4,867.65 |

figures are illustrative, but correspond well with other calculations made by the writer for specific premises. The figures for amortization of equipment are based on an autoscrubber costing approximately $2000, and a scrubber and suction-dryer costing together about $750, written off over five years. Table 5.9 is an attempt to summarize the relative numbers of cleaner-hours taken in maintaining various areas of floor, using:

1. Entirely manual methods (broom, mop with an efficient wringer)
2. A scrubber of the size specified, plus a 13 inch suction dryer
3. Autoscrubbers of the size specified.

These figures were compiled from experience in large factory areas, and do not allow for obstructions or any special jobs, such as stain removal. However, such matters would tend to increase the time taken whatever the method of cleaning.

**Table 5.9 Relative Speeds of Manual and Mechanical Floor Cleaning**

| Area (sq. ft.) | Manual | Scrubber + suction dryer | Autoscrubber |
|---|---|---|---|
| | | — — — — — — Man hours — — — — — — — — — — | |
| 2500 | 3 | 1 (15 in.) | 15 min (19 in.) |
| 5000 | 6 | 1½ (18 in.) | 24 min (21 in.) |
| 10,000 | 12 | 3 (18 in.) | 48 min (21 in.) |
| 15,000 | 18 | 4 (21 in.) | 72 min (21 in.) |
| 20,000 | 24 | 6 (21 in.) | i (26 in.) |
| 50,000 | 60 | 8 (30 in.) | 2½ (30 in.) |
| 100,000 | 120 | 16 (30 in.) | 5 (30 in.) |
| 200,000 | 240 | 32 (30 in.) | 7 (38 in.) |
| 500,000 | 600 | 80 (30 in.) | 7 (60 in.) |
| 1,000,000 | 1200 | 160 (30 in.) | 11 (72 in.) |

In this chapter the information on machines, etc., was kindly supplied by the following companies:

Advance Floor Machine Co., Spring Park, Minn. 55384

American Lincoln Co., Toledo, Ohio 43624

Atlas Floor Machinery Corp., 15 Jefferson St.,West Hartford,Conn. 06110

Billy Goat Industries Inc., P.O. Box 229, 12820 7th St., Grandview, Mo. 64030

Breuer Electric Mfg. Co., Chicago, Ill. 60640

Clarke Floor Machines, 30 East Clay Ave., Muskegon, Mich. 49443

Floorola Division, Hadco Corp., Center and Spruce Sts., Cleveland, Ohio 44113

Geerpress Wringer Co., P.O. Box 658, Muskegon, Mich. 49443

General Floorcraft Inc., 3630 Rombouts Ave., Bronx, New York, N.Y. 10466

Hild Floor Machine Co. Inc., 5339 W. Lake St., Chicago, Ill. 60644

National Super Service Co., Toledo, Ohio 43624

Nobles Industries Inc., 645 E 7th St., St. Paul, Minn. 55106

Somerset Power Sweepers, Route 219, South Somerset, Pa. 15501

Tennant Co., 721 Lilac Drive, Minneapolis, Minn. 55440

White Mop Wringer Co., Fultonville, N.Y. 12072

World Floor Machine Co., 2613 4th St. E, Minneapolis, Minn. 55414

All inquiries should be addressed to the companies listed above.

# PART II

# Specific Cleaning and Maintenance Procedures

# six

# Floors

Of all the surfaces in any type of building, the floor provides the greatest number and variety of cleaning and maintenance problems. Floors are, by their nature, constantly exposed to heavy loads, impact, abrasion, spills, and the action of dirt and moisture. It is only too often, as any maintenance manager knows to his chagrin, that the effect of one day's traffic in wet weather can effectively nullify the previous maintenance work of weeks. Add to this physical vulnerability the safety problems brought about by a littered, slippery, infectious or damaged floor surface, and it can easily be seen why floors are a major item in the planning and costing of any maintenance program. It has been calculated that at least one-third of the total time spent in cleaning and maintenance is expended on the care of floors (The American Hotel and Motel Association calculate 40 per cent for their buildings), and in hospitals, food stores and other places where absolute hygiene is necessary for health as well as esthetic reasons, the proportion may be even higher.

Despite this, it is a regrettable fact that these considerations enter too little into the discussions leading to the selection of flooring for new buildings. The architect is deeply concerned with the appearance, the heating engineer with the insulation properties, the structural engineer with the load-bearing capacity; but the ease, difficulty, or sometimes the impossibility of keeping the floor clean, whole, and safe is not considered until too late, usually by bitter experience. For this reason, this chapter has been written on the assumption that the maintenance manager already has certain types of flooring in his premises, and has to do the best he can with them. Each type of floor surface is dealt with under a separate heading, with notes on the advantages and disadvantages for various types of traffic and use, and recommendations for the most effective maintenance procedures.

At the same time, enough detail has been included, it is hoped, to assist in the selection of suitable surfaces for new buildings, or for the re-laying of existing floors, both inside and outside.

## TYPES OF FLOOR SURFACE

It is possible to classify types of floor surface in many different ways. They may, for instance, be grouped according to chemical type, so that metal, concrete, brick and stone floors would all be classified as mineral, and wood, linoleum, and synthetic plastic floors as organic. But this causes difficulties in dealing with concrete that has been modified with latex or synthetic resin binders, for instance, and thus are mineral *and* organic. Floors may be grouped as external or internal types, but asphalt, a very useful outdoor surface, is also used for many indoor applications, and conversely the demand for decorative architectural features has brought many "interior" types of flooring, such as terrazzo, into the open air. Therefore floorings have been divided, rather loosely, into heavy-duty types—suitable for conditions of trucking and wheeled traffic, heavy impact, spillage of chemicals and other reactive materials— and medium-duty types, suitable for normal foot traffic and light wheeled traffic.

HEAVY-DUTY FLOORINGS

### Concrete

This ubiquitous flooring material is a complex mixture of calcium aluminates and silicates (derived from the Portland cement component), sand, and various types of aggregate. It is cheap and hard-wearing, but is chemically attacked by acids, alkalis, and animal or vegetable fats and oils. The "floating" of a concrete surface to make it smooth and level tends to bring to the top a good deal of cement, known as "laitance," and this can be the cause of dustiness for months or even years after the floor has been laid. The older treatment to bind the dust on such a surface was to apply a solution of sodium silicate, either in the form of "water-glass" or as various proprietary mixtures. These bound down the laitance as calcium silicate. This is a cheap method of sealing, but the effect does not last more than a few weeks, and a better approach is to apply some of the newer organic seals. These can be oleoresinous materials like tung oil, which can be used in the form of a varnish or pigmented to make a floor paint, chlorinated rubber in a suitable solvent (with plasticizers to give the chlorinated rubber extra spreading power and elasticity), polyacrylate emulsions, or polyurethane sealers. Polyacrylates not only prevent dustiness but really seal the surface against the penetration of oil and oily dirt, thus saving much subsequent cleaning effort. Polyurethane seals, especially the two-can type, are more expensive but give a tougher surface than any of the other seals, and the surface is resistant to a wide variety of chemicals.

Polyurethane floor finishes will be mentioned under many of the headings in this chapter, so this may be an appropriate place to describe the products in more detail. Urethanes are organic chemicals formed when isocyanates react with alcohols. If each half of the partnership has more than one reacting group, the reaction produces chains or groups of urethane molecules, called *polyurethanes*, having the characteristics of a tough plastic material. The reaction can be carried out by the manufacturer of the polyurethanes, who is then selling the plastic material ready-formed, or it can be carried out by the user actually on the surface to be treated, in which case the isocyanate half and the alcohol half have to be packed separately, as in the epoxide adhesives that are widely sold. For obvious reasons the "ready-made" polyurethanes are called "one-can" types, and the others "two-can" types.

One-can polyurethanes are either "moisture cure" resins, where the final stages of setting are brought about by atmospheric moisture after the product has been spread over the floor, or oil-modified resins, which contain catalytic driers and set rather like a paint. Two-can polyurethanes usually contain a suitable isocyanate in one can, and a polyalcohol in the other. The usage of the various types may be judged from the 1967 sales figures: about 11 million gallons of polyurethanes were sold, of which 45-50 per cent were oil-modified types, 30-35 per cent moisture-cure types, 10 per cent two-can coatings, and the rest special types used for wire coating and similar purposes.

Once the concrete floor is sealed adequately, regular cleaning should consist of daily sweeping, followed when necessary by washing with neutral detergent and water. Alkali-built detergents should be avoided for regular use because of their damaging effect on the floor, and soap-based products avoided because they will produce a slippery surface of calcium soap that is a real safety hazard. In general a nonionic detergent is to be recommended, especially when used with floor machines.

The effective life of the floor seal can be extended greatly by following this regular washing with a polyacrylate or polyurethane type of floor polish, or, for greater resistance, a metallized emulsion polish. To avoid too great a build-up of polish, this "touching up" can be carried out with a diluted solution, applied thinly. Patching of this kind is quite feasible with modern polishes.

## Concrete Tiles or Flags

These form a ready-cast concrete floor, supplied in units from 4 inches to 18 inches square, and usually 5/8 inches to 1 ½ inches deep. Because they are manufactured under stricter control than is possible on a building site, they usually have a better dust-free surface. Mottled, grooved, and checker finishes are available, and some simple colors. They should be laid in cement mortar, cured for three to four days after laying. The maintenance treatment is the same as that for solid concrete. Although sealing is not essential, it will save a great deal of cleaning by preventing the penetration of grease and dirt.

## Monolithic Concrete Paving

In this flooring surface, the upper layer of a concrete slab floor is fed with specialized aggregates—granite chips, quartz or metal particles—which are exposed to form a bearing surface. This makes a surface resistant to abrasion, impact, water, frost, heat, alkalis, mineral oil and solvents, but like all concrete it is sensitive to acids, sulfates, and animal and vegetable oils and fats. Maintenance is the same as for plain concrete.

## Metal-Clad Flags

These are made in the same way as concrete flags, but a surface layer of steel chips is incorporated in the bearing surface while the concrete is setting. They are very resistant to trucking, abrasion, severe impact, and heat. The flags are usually laid on a concrete base, sometimes on sand or gravel, with a bed of 1:3 cement mortar, and buttered with Portland cement paste, followed by a cement paste grouting after 24 hours. Maintenance is the same as for concrete, except that seals are not usually applied. However, as a once-and-for-all operation, use of a seal will extend the life of the grouting.

## Granolithic

This is a specialized concrete finish made with cement, granite chips, sharp sand and/or granite dust. It can be applied by monolithic addition to a concrete subfloor (laying the granolithic coating within three hours of casting the main concrete slab), and in this case ½ inch to one inch thickness is satisfactory. Alternatively, it can be applied as a later addition to a set concrete subfloor, in which case one to two inches will be needed. It forms a drag-free, highly resistant floor which can stand static loading up to 7000 lb./in$^2$. Like all concrete bases it is attacked by acids, fats and oils, but some increased acid-resistant types are made by using high-alumina cement. The surface of granolithic floors is slippery unless abrasive powder is included in the face. Maintenance is the same as for plain concrete floors.

### Asphalt Cement (Bituminous Cement)

All the concrete floors considered up to now have the common disadvantages of concrete from the point of view of the comfort of the personnel using the floor: concrete is hard, cold, noisy, and often slippery, especially when wet. Asphalt cement is one of a class of concretes designed to have a warmer and more resilient surface. The usual mixture of cement, sand, and aggregate is used, but it is gauged with asphalt emulsion instead of plain water, so that asphalt is incorporated intimately into the cement mix. Asphalt cement may be laid over concrete, wood, or metal, and has the advantage that it can take a feather edge without chipping. The surface thus formed is water-resistant, quiet, warm, and flexible. It tends to indent permanently under heavy static loads such as machinery, and is more affected by oils, fats, and acids than ordinary concrete.

Maintenance of asphalt cement should involve daily sweeping, followed when necessary with a neutral detergent wash. Soap-based and alkaline detergents should be avoided, and solvents (whether by themselves or in wax paste polishes) must be kept away from the surface, as they will leach out the asphalt. On a new asphalt cement surface no sealing will be necessary, but after some time the surface becomes impoverished and porous, and an oleoresinous seal or floor paint is then useful. The floor paints, available in a variety of colors, have the effect of covering up blemishes and improving the general appearance.

### Latex Cement

In place of asphalt, concrete may be gauged with an emulsion of natural (rubber) or synthetic latexes which give a surface resistant to water, oils, dilute acids, alkalis, and sulfates. Polyvinyl acetate emulsions give increased resistance to oils and greases at some loss to the water resistance. Maintenance procedures should be the same as for asphalt cement, except that the surface of most latex cements responds well to treatment with polyacrylate or metallized emulsion polish. Solvents and solvent-based materials like wax paste polishes should be avoided.

### Mastic Asphalt

This is a blend of bitumen asphalt with fillers such as granite dust or other minerals, spread hot and finished to give a smooth continuous surface, usually between 5/8 inch and 2 inches thick. This flooring is very quiet and warm, dust-free, resistant to impact, water, alkalis, acids, sulfates, and most other aqueous chemicals. It may indent permanently under a heavy static load, and is softened by oils, fats, solvents and heat (it is definitely not suitable for use with underfloor heating). Initial treatment of a new mastic asphalt floor should be carried out about a week after laying. The floor is washed with nonionic detergent at about ¼ ounce (of 100 per cent material) in 5 gallons of water, and rinsed thoroughly, followed by drying, preferably by suction. It is then treated with two coats (about 20 minutes apart) of an emulsion polish of the polyacrylate type, buffing after each coat with a floor machine. This will not only help to seal the floor, preventing any penetration of dirt into the asphalt surface, but will also go a long way towards obviating the slipperiness of an asphalt floor when wet. Routine maintenance should follow this pattern: daily sweeping, followed when necessary by washing with a neutral detergent, and a "touch-up" coat of acrylate polish where it is needed. Soap-based products should not be used at all on asphalt, and solvents in any form will damage the surface. In any case, the use of such products as wax pastes, which contain solvents, is also likely to increase the slip of a mastic asphalt floor.

Asphalt surfaces for roofs and basements are usually made with softer grades of mastic asphalt, less hard-wearing but more waterproof, and self-healing if cracks are caused by movements of the structure underneath. If there is any need to clean these surfaces, nonionic detergent is recommended.

### Pitchmastic

This is a similar flooring to mastic asphalt, made of coal-tar pitch mixed with sand, chalk, granite dust, and similar fillers. It is usually laid in thicknesses from 5/8-1 inch, according to the weight of the traffic. Like mastic asphalt it is warm, dust-free, quiet, resilient, and resistant to water, acids, and sulfates, with fair resistance to alkalis, impact, and abrasion. Its resistance to fats and oils is better than that of asphalt, but solvents are very damaging to pitchmastic floors. The finish may be polished, semi-matt, or exposed aggregate. A polished surface is applied by adding wax in small quantities while floating the surface during laying, semi-matt and matt finishes by rubbing in varying quantities and gauges of a substance such as fine basalt flour while the pitch is setting. The aggregate can be exposed to give a non-slip surface by machine buffing just after the pitch has set. Maintenance should follow the same procedure as for mastic asphalt, except of course that the matt surfaces will not require any polish.

## Composition Blocks

These blocks are a blend of mineral and organic types of flooring, and consist of cement, wood flour or sawdust, gypsum, and chalk, bound with linseed oil, other drying oils, or plastics such as PVC. They form a floor which is warm and quiet, non-slip, non-dusting, resistant to mineral oils, greases, animal or vegetable fats and oils, dilute acids and alkalis, but not very resistant to repeated wetting. The blocks bound with PVC are better in wet conditions.

Initial treatment should consist of sweeping, followed by washing with a nonionic detergent or a nonionic/anionic blend, followed by suction drying. This should be followed by two coats of emulsion polish, using the polyacrylate or metallized type. (For a first application, the extra cost of the metallized polish is negligible compared with the great increase in resistance imparted to the floor.) Regular maintenance should consist of daily sweeping, followed when necessary by washing and treatment with emulsion polish. Soap, soap-based cleansers, solvents, and polishes containing solvents should not be used on composition blocks.

## Bricks and Other Paving Materials

These familiar baked-clay blocks form a floor resistant to oils, fats, acids and alkalis, solvents, and most other chemicals, but are cold, noisy, and slippery when wet. Initial treatment should consist of sweeping, washing with a nonionic detergent at about ½ ounce (100 per cent material) in 5 gallons of water, and application of a seal when the floor is dry. Oleoresinous, polyacrylate, or polyurethane seals are suitable, but the extra cost of the synthetic materials will be more than repaid by the saving in subsequent maintenance. In addition, the polyurethane seal will make bricks much less slippery. With a properly sealed floor, day-to-day maintenance can be reduced to sweeping, wiping over spills, etc., with a sponge applicator wetted with synthetic detergent solution, and washing when necessary with synthetic detergent. Soap is not recommended on this type of surface as it increases the slip, but any liquid detergent should be satisfactory.

## Unglazed Tiles

Unglazed tiles (quarry tiles) are available in sizes varying from 4 inches x 4 inches (usually about ¾ inches thick) to 12 inches x 12 inches (in thicknesses from 1 inch to 2 inches). Their properties are similar to those of bricks: instead of a cement mortar and grouting, they may be fixed in a bituminous bedding, which will fasten them to almost any surface, including sheet metal. Maintenance treatment is as for bricks and paving materials. In the case of quarries fastened with bitumen, care should be taken never to use solvents or products containing solvents, as these will soften the bitumen and affect the adhesion of the tiles.

### Ceramic Fully Vitrified Tiles

These glazed tiles are available in a wide range of sizes from 4 inches x 4 inches up to about 10 inches by 10 inches, in thicknesses from 3/8 inch to 1 ½ inches (for vitrified tiles). All of them are highly resistant to water and most types of chemicals, except hydrofluoric acid and concentrated alkali.

Maintenance should consist of regular washing with synthetic detergent solution; soap is not recommended because it may aggravate the already slippery surface of a tiled floor. Alkaline detergents may be used to remove heavy soiling, but it should be remembered that the grouting of the tiles is not as resistant as the glazed surface of the tiles themselves, and for habitual use a neutral detergent is better.

### Magnesite

This flooring is a continuous slab of magnesium oxychloride with asbestos, cork, sand, wood flour, and so on as filling, made by mixing the fillers with dry powdered magnesium oxide and then wetting the mass with magnesium chloride solution. It forms a smooth, light-colored floor, which is quiet, comparatively warm, with good impact resistance, and not affected by mineral oil or other oils and fats. It also has the unusual property of being almost entirely spark-proof when struck, even with steel, which can be a serious consideration in some industries. The mixture can be trowelled onto any surface, concrete, planks, or metal, but in the last case the metal surface should be carefully rustproofed because of the corrosive effect of the chloride ions in the magnesite. New magnesite floors should be sealed, preferably with an oleoresinous product such as tung oil. This will make subsequent cleaning very much easier. Regular maintenance should consist of daily sweeping, washing with synthetic detergent solution, and application of a polyacrylate emulsion polish. For the removal of heavy staining, a solvent-detergent blend may be quite useful; solvents are quite permissible on this type of floor. Alkaline products and soap should be avoided.

### Epoxy Resins

Epoxides can be polymerized under the influence of various catalysts, usually amines or peroxides, to form very tough, rigid plastics. When filled with glass fiber these form the familiar fiberglass construction material; filled with mineral dust and similar materials, they make a flooring notable for its high resistance to impact, weights, water, acids, fats, oils and alkalis. The epoxy resin is spread over the subfloor (concrete, asphalt, timber or metal) in thicknesses of 1/16 inch to ½ inch; to ensure proper adhesion to concrete, the laitance should be removed by acid etching before the resin is applied. Epoxy resin floors do not need sealing, and maintenance can be limited to daily sweeping followed by washing with synthetic detergent and water when necessary, and occasional polishing with a polyacrylate emulsion polish or treatment with a floor paint of this type. For heavy deposits or stains, alkaline detergents or solvent-detergent blends can be used with impunity.

### Polyester Resins

These materials share most of the properties of the epoxy resin, though they are less chemically resistant. They are, however, more resilient, and therefore better adapted for use under conditions of constant vibration. The load-bearing capacity is somewhat lower than that of epoxy resins, so polyesters should be spread thicker for extreme conditions. Maintenance procedures are similar to those for epoxy resin floors.

### Polyurethane Resins

Details of the formation of polyurethanes have already been given; when these are to be used as an actual flooring, not just a sealer, the resin is mixed with sand, asbestos, and other fillers. Polyurethanes are very hard yet very resilient, so their resistance to trucking, impact, and abrasion is equal to that of the polyester or epoxy resin floors, but they stand up better to strains induced by movements of the sub-floor and they have excellent non-skid properties. They are spread by floating or squeegee on concrete, hardboard, wood, steel, or aluminum floors, usually at about 1/16 inch thickness, or even thinner in the form of a non-skid paint, and finished by smoothing with a trowel dipped in solvent.

Maintenance of a polyurethane resin floor is very simple because of its high resistance to water, acids, alkalis, oils, fats, and other chemicals. Procedures are similar to those for epoxy resin floors.

### End-Grain Wood Blocks

Heavy-duty flooring can be formed from wood blocks if they are arranged to present an end-grain face on the bearing surface. They are usually 2 ½ inches or 5 inches deep, and are grouted with bituminous emulsion or melted pitch. Such a floor is warm, resilient, and has excellent sound deadening and heat insulating properties.

For industrial use a wood floor must be well sealed, but it is unwise to apply one of the conventional sealers directly to a new floor. Wood blocks tend to contract as they come into equilibrium with their surroundings, especially if underfloor heating is used. While the contraction of each individual block is very small and the gaps thus produced are hardly visible, the use of the tung oil type of seal, for instance, may bind large numbers of blocks together in such a way that the contraction only appears as cumulative large gaps at the edges of groups of many blocks. This shrinkage may take six to twelve months, and obviously the floor must be protected in some way during this time. Specialized priming coats have been developed for this purpose, which protect the wood without sticking the blocks together too tightly. Over this primer a tougher seal can be applied, using the oleoresinous (tung oil) type, polyacrylates, or polyurethanes. A one-can urea-formaldehyde resin is also suitable. The type of traffic and the materials handled must indicate the final choice.

Regular maintenance of a sealed wood floor requires daily sweeping and removal of spilled materials with a damp cloth, followed by spraying or mopping when necessary with a water-based emulsion polish, either of the polyacrylate type or, for really hard conditions, a metallized type. Wax polish may be used, but once the floor has been started on this treatment it is difficult to change, and the labor requirement will be found much greater than with "dry-bright" polishes. If a floor is already treated with a wax polish and a change of method is desired, thorough stripping of the wax is the only solution. A section on stripping floors is given at the end of this chapter.

## Metal Anchor Plates and Metal Paving Tiles

These metal floors present the most resistant finishes of all. Metal anchor plates are made of steel with projecting anchors or grips. They are laid on a concrete surface in a stiff bedding of 1 part cement, 2 parts sand, 1 ½ parts gravel, buttered with a cement grout and butted.

Metal paving tiles are iron castings with shallow feet, which are bedded down in cement and worked down until the feet touch the concrete sub-floor.

Both these floor finishes are cold and noisy, but they display outstanding resistance to trucking, impact, abrasion, heat, vibration, oils, fats and alkalis. Maintenance is limited to washing with detergent solution with or without added alkali, according to the degree of soiling. Soap products should not be used because they make the metal slippery.

## Jointing Compounds

As so many of the heavy-duty finishes depend on cement of some kind for jointing and grouting, it may be useful to summarize the main types of such jointing compounds and their resistance to various types of chemical. Table 6.1 is such a summary.

MEDIUM DUTY FLOORINGS

## Marble, Natural Stone

The care of marble and other natural stone in flooring is usually associated with the upkeep of historic or "prestige" buildings, where the preservation and appearance of the floor are of prime importance, and damage may be very costly to repair and almost impossible to tone to the original. Therefore, although these floorings are very resistant to certain types of traffic, they are classified as medium-duty, along with the other decorative types of floor. Marble and most natural stones are particularly sensitive to the action of aicds, which will etch them and permanently damage the surface, and, to a lesser extent, alkalis, which may penetrate the natural grain of the stone and cause swelling, with flaking, cracking, and even lifting of the stones as a consequence. It is important to ensure that all cleaning materials are neutral. A nonionic or blended anionic/nonionic detergent may be used with safety, but soaps, soap powders and built detergent powders should be strictly avoided. Stone floors may be sealed and polished by the application of thin coats of emulsion polish (polyacrylate or polyurethane) followed by buffing, and this will help to minimize the slippery nature of a marble floor. Wax-based polishes will increase the slip, and should not be used.

## Terrazzo

This flooring is made up of chips of colored marble or similar decorative stone set, mosaic-fashion, in white cement. It thus combines the qualities of a marble floor and a high-quality concrete floor. Terrazzo may be laid in one continuous slab, or it may be made of "tiles" of terrazzo in contrasting shades or textures. Like its components, terrazzo is sensitive to acids and alkalis, and its porous nature makes it particularly subject to absorbing greasy dirt as a permanent stain. To obviate this, the following initial treatment is recommended. Scrub with a neutral detergent, preferably of the nonionic type; if the floor has become very soiled during building operations, scrubbing with fine pumice powder or commercial scourer may be necessary, followed by a detergent wash and wet pick-up of the rinsings. Rinse thoroughly in any case with clean water and leave to dry, or dry mechanically. Then apply a thin coat of emulsion

**Table 6.1 Resistance of Jointing Compounds to Various Agents**

| Jointing compound | Water | Organic acids | Hydrochloric acid | Sulfuric acid | Nitric acid | Caustic alkali | Sulfates | Mineral oil | Vegetable oil | Organic solvents |
|---|---|---|---|---|---|---|---|---|---|---|
| Portland cement mortar | vg | p | vp | vp | vp | g | p | g | p | g |
| Supersulfate mortar | vg | g | f | f | f-p | g | g | g | g | g |
| High alumina mortar | vg | g | vp | vp | vp | f | g | g | f | g |
| Silicate cement | p | g | g | g | g | vp | g | g | g | g |
| Sulfur cement | vg | g | g | g | f | g | g | g | p | g |
| Phenol-formaldehyde resin | vg | g | g | f | p | g | g | g | g | f |
| Cashew nut resin | vg | g | g | f | p | g | g | p | p | p |
| Furan resin | vg | g | g | g | f | vg | g | g | g | g |
| Epoxy resin | vg | f | g | g | f | vg | g | g | f | f |
| Polyester resin | vg | g | g | g | f | p | g | g | g | f |
| Polyurethane resin | vg | g | g | g | f | p | g | g | g | f |

vg = very good, g = good, f = fair, p = poor, vp = very poor polish of the acrylate type and buff. This treatment may have to be repeated after 20 minutes if the floor appears to be very porous. Such pretreatment will repay the trouble several times over, as it will effectively seal a terrazzo floor against the penetration of dirt and grease, and subsequent regular maintenance can be limited to daily sweeping, washing as necessary with neutral liquid detergent solution, and reapplication, every month or so, of a coating of acrylate emulsion polish. On no account should soaps or built detergent powders be used on a terrazzo floor. If in doubt, it is better to avoid all powdered cleansers and use plain liquid detergent.

## Wood

Wood, in the form of strips or parquet blocks, is one of the commonest forms of interior flooring. It is warm, resilient, has good sound insulation properties, and can have a most attractive appearance when properly maintained. The disadvantage is that wood is porous, and likely to swell or distort when exposed to water.

The older treatment for wood was the application of so-called button polish and wax. Button polish, a solution of shellac in alcohol, is a fairly satisfactory sealer, but the maintenance of the wax finish is an expensive process, and on a new floor the following procedure is to be preferred. Assuming the wood surface has been sanded to a fine finish, remove dust by vacuum cleaning. Do not wash unless the floor is exceptionally dirty, as the use of water at this stage will only raise the grain of the wood and undo the effect of the sanding. If washing is absolutely necessary, the use of a scrubbing machine with a controlled water applicator is recommended. If the wood floor is a new block floor, apply one coat of a specially formulated primer, as the use of a stronger seal may cause cumulative movement of the blocks (see the section on end-grain wood blocks, p.142). After this pretreatment of the blocks, or directly on established floors, apply a seal. This should be selected according to the type of traffic and treatment anticipated. Oleoresinous sealers of the tung oil type are very effective for most purposes. Apply the seal freely in a first coat, working with the grain of the wood and avoiding overlapping as far as possible. Allow this coat to dry for about four hours, more or less according to the ambient temperature. Then apply a second, thinner coat of seal, finishing smooth (an applicator, as supplied by many of the manufacturers of seals, is useful here) and leave this to dry for 24 hours. Maintain a free circulation of air by opening windows, etc.

More expensive but harder wearing seals are made from urea-formaldehyde resins; application is carried out in the same way as for tung oil seals.

For the greatest resistance to traffic and chemicals, a "two-can" polyurethane seal should be used. These are still more expensive than the seals previously mentioned, but they produce a surface so hard that subsequent maintenance is reduced to a minimum. Shortly before use, a solution containing the isocyanate component is mixed with a solution containing the polyester resin. This produces a polyurethane resin on the spot. The manufacturers' instructions must be followed implicitly, because the ingredients must be mixed thoroughly without undue delay in spreading (obviously the resin will set eventually whether it is on the floor or still in the can; this means that the work must be carried out more carefully than with the "paint" type of finish that only sets when exposed to air).

A floor so treated can be maintained regularly by daily sweeping, followed by light spraying or mopping with emulsion polish whenever necessary to restore the gloss. This method of treatment avoids the use of excessive amounts of water, which can raise the grain of the wood, and if the floor is buffed while the polish is still damp, a fine finish can be obtained.

Similar maintenance procedures are suitable for floors of reconstituted wood. These consist of wood chips and wood flour bound together by a plastic resin. Usually the resin is very resistant to penetration by water, and less trouble need be taken in sealing the surface initially.

## Cork

This flooring forms one of the most quiet, comfortable and warm surfaces on which to work. Cork granules are compressed into sheets or tiles, usually with a binder, and baked to aggregate the mass. The great disadvantage of cork is that the surface is extremely porous, and takes up dirt, grease, and moisture to a far greater extent than wood. The sealing methods given for the initial treatment of wood floors are all eminently suitable for cork, and the need to carry them out is even more stringent. For regular maintenance of a cork floor, the best procedure is daily sweeping followed by a very light spraying with emulsion polish, preferably of the polyacrylate type, and buffing while the polish is still damp. If a wax polish is preferred, there are special filler polishes that can be rubbed into the surface, left for an hour or two to dry, and then buffed with a nylon or steel wool pad.

## Linoleum

This is a mixture of cork flour, wood flour, pigment, and other fillers, bound with linseed and similar drying oils and resin. The mixture is backed with burlap or felt. It may be laid down from the continuous roll, or in the form of linoleum tiles, stuck onto a smooth underfloor. The surface is not as continuous or impervious as it may look to the naked eye, and some kind of initial sealing is just as necessary for linoleum as for cork. A urea-formaldehyde seal is recommended. With many varieties of linoleum, especially in the roll form, the makers apply a dressing to protect and give gloss to the surface during store-life, and this may interfere with the proper adhesion of the seal; it may be removed with a solvent/detergent cleanser.

The regular maintenance of linoleum may be carried out by daily sweeping and occasional application of emulsion polish. Linoleum should not be wetted too much or too often, as this tends to swell the cork granules. If it needs to be washed thoroughly, a neutral detergent should be used, avoiding soap, soap-based powders, and detergent powders. Alkalis in these powders, sometimes present in large proportion, will also tend to swell the cork and destroy the smoothness of the surface. This will lead to a deterioration in appearance, more costly maintenance, and frequently loss of color and pattern.

### Rubber

Natural and synthetic rubber forms a soft, quiet, and warm flooring material that can be produced in very attractive designs. The main disadvantages of rubber flooring are its sensitivity to oils, fats, greases and solvents, and the tendency of the fillers in the rubber to swell if exposed to alkalis. This breaks up the surface. Rubber floors should be sealed to avoid this. The floor, when newly laid, should be scrubbed with nonionic detergent, allowed to dry or dried with wet suction, and then given two coats of emulsion polish, buffing while the emulsion is slightly damp. On no account should wax paste or solvent-based products be used on rubber.

When the floor has been sealed, regular maintenance consists of daily sweeping, using a damp cloth or mop to wipe up spillage (a nonionic detergent can be used on difficult patches) and periodic application of an emulsion polish of the same sort that was used for the initial application. This can be sprayed just ahead of the buffing machine or mopped over in dilute form, and followed by the buffing machine.

When thorough washing is necessary avoid soaps and soap-based products, and also highly alkaline detergents. Provided the floor has been adequately sealed, powdered detergents of the general-purpose type can be used on rubber floors.

### Epoxy Resins, Polyester Resins, Polyurethane Resins

See the appropriate sections under heavy-duty floorings.

## Asphalt Tiles

These are asbestos or other mineral fillers bound with asphalt or resinous materials. They are produced in a wide range of colors and patterns, and can be used over almost any type of subfloor by proper selection of adhesive. The tiles are sensitive to solvents, and to some extent to oils and fats, and therefore solvent-based cleansers and wax paste polishes should be avoided. If possible, the amount of water used in cleaning these tiles should be limited (for instance, by using a floor machine with a controlled flow device for the detergent), not because the tiles themselves are sensitive to moisture, but because all too often the adhesive used to secure them is not sufficently water-resistant. Where it is known beforehand that conditions are going to be wet or the traffic is so dirty that frequent washing will be a necessity, the tile manufacturers should be consulted about the best adhesive for the conditions and their recommendations followed implicitly.

Maintenance of asphalt tiles follows the same lines as for rubber; the same sealing and polishing methods will maintain a fine finish.

## Vinyl Tiles

These are made in the same way as asphalt tiles, except that the binder is PVC. This material is one of the toughest and most resistant of the vinyl plastics, and tiles made from it are harder wearing than asphalt tiles. Maintenance follows the same lines as for rubber floors.

## STAIN REMOVAL

However well the floor is prepared and maintained, there will always be some time when an unusual degree of soiling baffles the cleaning staff, and emergency action becomes necessary. The following notes may be useful for dealing with one of these emergencies, although it should be stressed that most of these methods are for *occasional* use only, and some of them may cause slight damage to the surface. However, when serious staining occurs, it is often a choice between slight deterioration of the floor or leaving the stain on, with greater deterioration of the floor's appearance.

### CONCRETE

Because of its porous nature concrete tends to stain rather easily, and discoloration may go very deep. The following methods may be tried.

They will also apply to the cement portions of such floorings as terrazzo, the grouting of tiles, and other cement "trimmings."

### Iron Stains

These may be caused by water with rust in it from a deteriorating water tank, from the use of rusty water for curing the cement, or from condensation dripping from pipework, structural members, and so on. For large areas, make up a solution of one pound of oxalic acid (CAUTION— POISONOUS) to each gallon of water, spread it over the surface and leave it for three hours; rinse thoroughly and scrub with dilute detergent solution. This treatment should not be carried out on terrazzo, as the acid will etch the marble chips.

For bad iron stains in small spots, make up a solution of sodium citrate at about three ounces to a pint of water, mix the solution with an equal quantity of glycerin, and stir in whiting to make a paste. Apply this paste with a trowel, fairly thickly, and leave it to dry. Reapply if necessary. Similar treatment is suitable for terrazzo.

An alternative that will often clear up old iron stains that are resistant to normal treatment is to make up the sodium citrate solution as above (without the whiting), dip a sponge in the solution, and spread it over the stains. Leave them soaking for 15 minutes, then sprinkle the patches thinly with crystals of sodium hydrosulfite. Leave for a further one hour (not longer, otherwise black stains may develop) and wash off thoroughly. Scrub as before.

### Copper Stains

These stains may arise from condensation dripping from copper roofing, plumbing fixtures, or decorative bronzes and the like. They appear as dirty blue-green patches that are very resistant to cleaning. The best treatment is to make up one part of ammonium chloride (sal ammoniac), four parts talc or powdered chalk, and enough ammonia solution (ordinary household ammonia) to make a paste. Spread this paste over the stains and leave it to dry, then wash off carefully and scrub or brush.

### Ink Stains

Ink stains will usually yield to hydrogen peroxide or a solution of sodium perborate made up to a paste with whiting or powdered chalk. The action is faster if the paste is heated, and this can be done conveniently by spreading paper over the paste and applying an electric iron cautiously. If the ink is of the permanent type there may be a brown stain left after the peroxide treatment; treat this as for iron. Inks containing Prussian Blue (as some process inks) can be decolorized with ammonia water, as can the black stains left by marking ink.

### Lubricating Oil

These and similar oil stains may be removed by making up a solution of 1 ½ ounces trisodium phosphate to one pint of water, making this into a paste with whiting or powdered chalk. This paste should be spread over the stains. Heat, applied as above, is a great help with oil stains.

### Fire Stains

The brown stains left after a fire are very persistent and may be difficult to alter to any significant extent. They consist largely of tars generated by the fire, and penetrate concrete very deeply. The best treatment is to make up a paste with a solution of trisodium phosphate (two pounds to one gallon of water), one pint of sodium hypochlorite solution (at about 10 per cent available chlorine), and talc. Apply this paste with a trowel and leave it till it dries, then wash off. Several applications may be necessary if the concrete has been badly blackened.

### Rotten Wood

If wood has been allowed to lie on a concrete floor in damp conditions, it is quite likely that a brown stain will be left, and these stains are very permanent. Treat as for fire stains, except that one application of the paste will probably be sufficient.

### Iodine Stains

These sometimes occur in hospitals and sick bays. Alcohol will remove all but the heaviest stains, and is the safest material to use. Alternatively, a solution of three ounces of sodium thiosulfate to a pint of water, made up to a paste with talc, will bleach the stain. In emergency, photographers' fixer solution ("hypo") can be used.

### Urine Stains

These can be treated as for fire stains. One application of the paste should be sufficient.

### Crayon Marks

Those of the wax crayon type can be removed with acetone. This solvent is quite safe to handle apart from being flammable. It will also remove *lipstick* and *nail polish* from concrete.

## Paint

This should be removed with one of the solvent type paint strippers. These are based on methylene chloride thickened with a synthetic gum such as methylcellulose. Spread the stripper thickly over the paint, scrape as the paint is softened, remove as much as possible of the paint and stripper with a squeegee or the edge of a trowel, and wash with water.

## Bloodstains

Bloodstains can be removed with sodium hypochlorite solution at two per cent available chlorine. If the normal 10 per cent material is purchased, one pint should be diluted with four pints of water. Always use cold water when removing bloodstains. If a brown stain remains after the hypochlorite treatment, remove this as for iron stains.

### GLAZED TILES

Glazed tiles are usually very resistant to staining, but sometimes soiling seems very adherent. The following brief list of remedies represents a reasonable solution for some common troubles; many of these are the same as for concrete, and details of their preparation or use will be found in the previous section.

*Iron, rust:* one part sodium citrate, seven parts glycerin, talc or whiting to make a paste; apply thickly.

*Copper, bronze:* one part ammonium chloride, one part household ammonia, talc to make a paste.

*Ink:* sodium hypochlorite solution, 1:4 diluted with water. If a brown stain remains, treat as for iron.

*Marking ink and Prussian Blue ink:* wash with household ammonia.

*Ballpoint pen ink:* wash with alcohol or acetone.

*Oil:* wash with gasoline, or use a solution of two ounces of trisodium phosphate to one pint of water, made to a paste with talc or whiting.

*Paint:* use methylene chloride, trichloroethylene or commercial paint stripper.

*Crayon, lipstick nail polish:* use acetone.

*Blood:* wash with sodium hypochlorite solution, 1:4 with water.

*Shoe polish:* use white spirit.

### WOOD, CORK, LINOLEUM

These surfaces are not likely to be affected by iron or copper stains, but the removal of stains such as blood, coffee, or tea, may cause difficulties. The following treatments are recommended.

## Coffee and Tea Stains

These may be removed by sodium hypochlorite solution or a paste made up with hypochlorite and talc. It is inevitable that some bleaching of the wood and linoleum will take place, but with a dilute solution (about 1 per cent available chlorine, i.e. normal 10 per cent bleach diluted 1:9 with water) it should be possible to decolorize the stain before the wood, or the color of the linoleum, is greatly affected. In cases of this kind, the very real value of proper sealing will be appreciated, because a well-sealed floor does not stain easily.

Similar treatment will remove *bloodstains* and ordinary *inkstains.*

## Marking Ink

This can be removed with diluted household ammonia, about 1:4 with water.

After any of these treatments, the floor should be washed thoroughly and then resealed by the application of polyacrylate polish.

## MAGNESITE

Magnesite floors are very resistant to most inorganic stains, such as rust and copper, and to spilling in general. It is worth remembering that magnesite is quite resistant to solvents, and therefore oil, tar, rubber heel marks, and similar "greasy" stains can be removed with white spirit from this type of flooring. Gasoline can be used in emergency, with proper fire precautions.

## VINYL TILES

Vinyl tiles are not likely to become stained to any depth, especially if they are properly sealed, but stains that are resistant to washing can often be removed by the addition of dilute sodium hypochlorite to the washing water (domestic bleach 1:9 with detergent solution). This treatment will brighten the surface of white tiles that are becoming a little discolored. After treatment, the floor should be resealed.

## STRIPPING OF FLOORS

In all cases where treatment is recommended with emulsion or wax polishes, there will come a time when the build-up of polish on the floor is itself unsightly. Modern products are formulated to avoid most of the yellowing that is associated with shellac and similar materials, but it still occurs to some extent, and in several coats of polish, laid one over another, the effect is dulling. More serious is the gradual incorporation of dirt into the polish layer, which causes darkening. About twice a year (more or less, according to the traffic and conditions in the particular area) the old coats of polish should be stripped off and a new start made.

Wax, polystyrene and polyacrylate polishes can be stripped by going over the surface with a hot solution of nonionic detergent at about 1 per cent concentration of active detergent. If the detergent is bought at the common concentration of about 25 per cent, then a solution of about 1/3 pint per gallon is appropriate. A scrubbing machine fitted with nylon floor cleaning pads will do the job quickly and efficiently (the use of steel wool pads is likely to leave small rusty fragments on the floor). Thorough scrubbing should be followed by rinsing and drying. In the case of wood, cork and other moisture-sensitive floorings, the amount of detergent solution should be limited as far as possible. This also applies to vinyl and asphalt tile surfaces if there is any doubt about the stability of the adhesive to water, as the penetrating effect of hot detergent solution will tend to aggravate any water-seepage under the tiles.

Metallized emulsion polishes, which are more resistant to abrasion and ordinary cleansers, will not be stripped by the above treatment. They need a detergent solution containing ammonia. All the suppliers of such polishes supply a suitable stripping compound. Alternatively, the following mixture may be made up:

| | |
|---|---|
| Nonionic detergent (25 per cent active detergent) | ½ pint |
| Household ammonia | ¼ pint |
| Hot water | 1 gallon |

After stripping, all floors should be re-primed with two coats of the chosen polish. It is useful to finish off the second coat at right angles to the first, as this helps to avoid heavy overlap lines and covers up any gaps left in the first coat.

If it is desired to remove old wax polishes and replace them by a more modern type, it is particularly important that all the wax is removed, otherwise the emulsion polish will not adhere properly. Two effective methods are as follows:

1. Use a solvent-detergent mixture (not on rubber, asphalt tiles, vinyl tiles, or similar solvent-sensitive floors) and a medium nylon scrubbing pad.
2. Spray the surface, a little at a time, with liquid polish, and scrub immediately with a coarse nylon pad.

In either case the pads will become saturated with wax after a while; they can be washed out in a bucket of white spirit at intervals.

# seven

# Interiors, Walls and Windows

In addition to the dirt and debris brought into buildings on shoes, on the wheels of vehicles, and the like, there is a constant silent invasion of dust. Soot and dirt from fires and furnaces, mineral dust eroded away from rocks by wind and rain, blown soil, textile fragments from the imperceptible breaking down of clothes and furnishing, pollen, seeds, gum and other plant fragments, all contribute to the clouds of dust that we take for granted as a fact of existence. The number of particles of dust in the atmosphere will obviously vary according to the surroundings. In a town with heavy industry, for example, there may be a million or more particles per cubic foot of air, while high up over a large ocean the number may be as low as 250 per cubic foot, mostly salt particles and volcanic dust. The following figures (Table 7.1) have been quoted as typical of:

1. Open country (rural)
2. A small town with light industry, but no particularly "dirty" industries (urban)
3. A machine shop in full production.

The sizes of the particles have been given in microns ($\mu$) = one millionth of a millimeter.

**Table 7.1 Dust Contents of Various Samples of Air**

| Average size of particles ($\mu$) | Particles per ft.$^3$ | | |
|---|---|---|---|
| | Rural | Urban | Machine shop |
| 0.7-1.4 | 35,000 | 1,325,000 | 2,122,000 |
| 1.4-2.8 | 13,500 | 122,000 | 113,000 |

**Table 7.1 (cont.)**

| Average size of particles $(\mu)$ | Particles per ft.$^3$ | | |
| --- | --- | --- | --- |
| | Rural | Urban | Machine shop |
| 2.8-5.6 | 4,500 | 39,000 | 5,000 |
| 5.6-11.2 | 1,100 | 3,500 | 1,700 |
| 11.2-22.4 | — — | 550 | 500 |
| Totals | 54,100 | 1,490,050 | 2,242,200 |

The analysis of these particles of dust into various types of material, in the case of the urban sample, had the following results (Table 7.2):

**Table 7.2 Composition of Dust in Town Air**

| Type of material | Percentage |
| --- | --- |
| Sand, clay, quartz, feldspar | 45 |
| Limestone, dolomite | 5 |
| Animal fibers (wool, hair etc.) | 12 |
| Gypsum, apatite | 5 |
| Cellulose (cotton and paper fibers, plant debris) | 12 |
| Resins, gums, starches | 10 |
| Fats, oils, rubber, tar | 6 |
| Moisture | 3 |
| Undetermined | 2 |

Until recent years, it had been taken for granted that these particles cannot be kept out of premises, and the only remedy has been to dust, sweep, and vacuum them up when they get too noticeable. However, the growth of such industries as the manufacture of micro-electronic circuits and miniaturized apparatus of all kinds has brought about a new attitude towards dust. One speck of dust can ruin certain types of electronic apparatus, and the normal workroom atmosphere with up to two million particles per cubic foot is quite out of the question for these industries. In the hospital field, also, there has been a demand for wards that can be freed from the usual hazard of airborne bacteria, so that patients can be subjected to complex surgery without a consequently increased risk of infection.

The two demands have come together in the development of the "white room" and the aseptic ward. It is outside the scope of this book to discuss the immense medical problems of maintaining an aseptic ward, but white rooms have become important in many industries and may be expected to become more common in the future. For example, there is evidence that some of the costly breakdowns in computers may be due to dust contamination, and there is a demand for white rooms in which to house these expensive pieces of equipment.

A white room can be defined as a space in which air-borne contamination, and usually temperature and humidity, are controlled to a degree far higher than that in normal air-conditioned rooms. By definition, the dust in a white room should never exceed 100,000 particles ($0.5\mu$ in size or larger), and 700 particles ($5\mu$ in size or larger). The conditions are therefore more stringent than those in the open country quoted in Table 7.1.

Sources of dust in a room are manifold:

1. External dust penetrating the air-conditioning system;
2. Flaking and dusting from walls, floors, and ceilings;
3. Moving equipment, especially drills, polishers, and other machinery producing dust or chips;
4. Dust produced by the air conditioning equipment itself (fan blades, electric motors and so on) and compressed air supply if it is provided;
5. Human beings: skin, hairs, dandruff, saliva, makeup;
6. Textiles: clothes, wiping cloths, curtains;
7. Pencils, paper, erasers;
8. Smoking, eating;
9. Dust on parts brought in for manufacture.

The obvious first step is to eliminate as many as possible of these sources. Smoking and eating are forbidden, and glazed paper and ballpoint pens provided for writing, instead of pencils and erasers. All personnel wear lint-free coveralls and head covering, with clean shoes or overshoes, so that particles from their bodies are at least confined, even if they cannot be prevented from detaching themselves.

A typical large white room is that used by the North American Rockwell Space Research Division, where the following precautions represent some of the ways of overcoming the difficulties of maintaining such a high standard of cleanliness.

Employees, on entering the outer regions of the room, pass through an "air shower," in which a 30 m.p.h. jet of clean air sweeps downwards over them and through a perforated floor and filter system. While they are being dusted in this way, their shoes are cleaned by a mechanical doormat which scrubs the soles and polishes the uppers. They then put on special lintless coveralls and head covering, and PVC boots over their normal shoes. Finally they are admitted to the room itself through an airlock.

All parts and equipment come into the room through similar air showers. Small parts are encased in plastic bags if they have to be taken from one room to another through the "outside." The room itself is specially designed to be as free as possible from dust, or any materials that flake, crack, or powder. Welding is forbidden, and drilling is carried out by two people, one to use a slow speed drill and the other to pick up the drillings with a vacuum cleaner immediately. Cleaning goes on continually throughout every work period, so as to reduce any dust which has gotten in despite the precautions. A centralized vacuum cleaner system takes most of the dust, but surfaces are also dusted with "tack cloths" impregnated with rubber latex, polyvinyl acetate, or acrylics, as the sticky substance.

Personnel are, understandably, given a 15-hour training program to explain the reasons for the precautions, and to illustrate the seriousness of the losses that may occur if dust is allowed into the room through carelessness.

Apart from these particular precautions, the room itself is engineered to make them work properly. Air coming into the room is filtered to stop any particles over $0.5\ \mu$ and the room is kept at a slight positive pressure (0.5-1.0 inch of water) so that there is no chance of dirty air being sucked in from the outside. Whenever an airlock opens, air goes out, not in. All surfaces are smooth and free from sharp corners, and all can be washed. There are no textiles except the clothing of the personnel.

While the operation of such a white room is not necessary for many industries, some of the lessons of the system can be applied in a modified form in ordinary plants and offices. Air conditioning, for example, not only makes for a pleasanter environment, but greatly reduces the amount of dust and dirt which penetrates into premises, and therefore reduces the cleaning and maintenance costs—a point often overlooked when the costs of air conditioning are being discussed. Employees in the ordinary office may not be subjected to a 30 m.p.h. air shower, but they can be prevented from tracking in dust on their shoes by the installation of really effective doormats. Too often doormats are so small that people step over them, or they are allowed to become so dirty that they themselves become sources of dirt in the building.

With coconut fiber mats, the weight of the foot tends to compress the fiber and thus reduce its absorptive powers. When weather is wet the mat becomes soggy. It takes very little time for such a mat to become saturated with dirt, which can dry and blow into the building.

Link mats, usually made of rubber (old automobile tires are often used, cut into strips) are somewhat better and retain sufficient edge, even under compression, to scrape the dirt from the soles of shoes. The main problem with these mats is that they have very little capacity for dirt.

A more modern approach is the "open-strip" or cavity mat, in which strips of synthetic rubber are held vertically by stainless steel wires in such a way that they act as squeegees against the sole of the shoe, flicking the dirt away and trapping it in a cavity, usually about one inch deep, between each strip. The mats fit into a special well which retains the dirt until it needs to be removed. Uses of such mats are very wide, from the usual sites at entrances of factories, schools, and offices, to whole floors or corridors made of cavity matting. Carpeted buildings such as theaters and concert halls will find a large area of cavity matting useful to prevent dirt getting on the carpet.

A source of dirt entering a building that is often overlooked is a blocked or saturated air-conditioning filter screen. These are usually out of sight and out of mind, but can often get to a condition where they add more dirt to the incoming air than it contained already.

Unless the manufacturers' instructions definitely forbid this, such filters can usually be cleansed by hosing with nonionic detergent in warm water.

Tack rags, used in white rooms, are also well worth introducing into ordinary cleaning and maintenance practice. Every housewife knows that a duster is worse than useless if it is merely used to flick dirt from one place to another; it must pick up the dirt. The tack rag makes it almost impossible to spread dust, and will repay its cost, compared with common dusters, by reducing the time taken in cleaning.

## WINDOWS

The cleaning of windows is not really more difficult than that of any other smooth surfaces, but any deficiencies in the results show up much more clearly, so standards have to be higher. Windows are commonly covered with a faint greasy layer composed of oil and rubber from automobiles, furnaces, and the like, and to this layer adhere all kinds of solid particles. The object of cleaning must be to remove the greasy layer and take the dust with it.

A window-cleaning product must have the following properties:

1. It must remove grease of all kinds;
2. It must suspend dust particles well;

3. It must contain no abrasives that could scratch the glass;
4. It must leave no residue that is visible either as opaque material or as streaks or greasy-looking marks.

The old-fashioned household window-cleaning product was a mixture of ammonia water and whiting. The ammonia helped to dissolve the grease without leaving the same solid residues as sodium carbonate or similar alkalis, and the whiting acted as a mild abrasive, not hard enough to scratch the glass but enough to detach any sticky dirt; it also helped to absorb the grease. The mixture was left to dry on the window, and the powdery whiting then polished off with a clean cloth. The whiting tended to act more as an encouragement to proper cleaning than as any really effective polishing agent.

Better results are obtained with water-soluble solvents such as Cellosolve (a trade mark for ethylene glycol monoethyl ether), which have the unusual properties of dissolving grease almost as well as chlorinated solvents, yet are themselves soluble in water. These materials, in solution, will remove the grease from windows and dissolve away in the rinsing water, leaving no visible residue. As the solvents are colorless, traces that are left on the glass cause no trouble.

Professional window cleaners tend to use water alone, relying on the frictional action of chamois leather or a sponge to remove the grease, but their results are often unsatisfactory, and the use of a solvent in the water would increase their productivity and efficiency. An alternative, or addition, to the solvent is a small amount of nonionic detergent, and really excellent results can be obtained with a cleaning solution consisting of 1/10 ounce nonionic detergent (at 25 per cent) and 1/10 ounce Cellosolve per gallon of water. If the following technique is used, the results should be very good.

1. Use a cellulose sponge, chamois, and a rubber squeegee. Instead of the chamois, another sponge may be used.
2. Prepare the solution described above.
3. Wet the glass with one sponge dipped in the solution, going all around the pane and finishing up by wiping the edges of the frame to pick up dirt that has been pushed against the sides.
4. Squeegee the glass before dry spots appear. With the squeegee tilted so that about two inches of the blade touches the glass, start at the top corner of the pane and draw the blade along the upper edge of the glass. Wipe the squeegee blade with the chamois or the other sponge. Now, with the squeegee flat against the glass for the whole length of the blade, draw it down from the dry area at the top nearly to the bottom of the pane; repeat this along the whole width. The strokes should overlap. Wipe the blade on the chamois or second sponge after every stroke.

5. Finish the strip along the bottom of the glass with the squeegee blade vertical. Dry the water from the frame with the sponge, taking care not to touch the glass.

The sequence of operations is illustrated in Figure 7.1; it takes longer to describe than to perform in practice.

Large windows such as store fronts can be divided into two parts: the top half is cleaned by "cutting the water" vertically with the squeegee at an angle, and then the cleaning strokes are made horizontally from this beginning. The lower half is then wetted and cleaned in the same way.

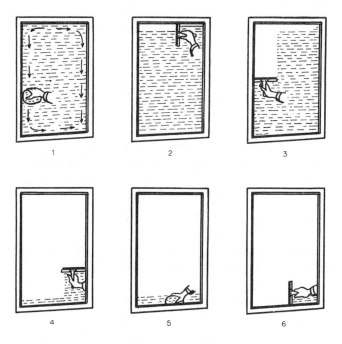

Figure 7.1

Window cleaning with a squeegee.

The preliminary action of "cutting the water" is to ensure that the squeegee starts from a clean dry surface. Squeegeeing of glass is like detergency in reverse. In detergency the detergent solution penetrates under the soiling and lifts it by having a greater affinity for the surface than the dirt. The squeegee has a greater affinity for dry glass than the washing solution has, and therefore if it can be given a small area of dry glass to start from, the detergent solution need never penetrate under the squeegee blade. It is very important to wipe the squeegee blade after every stroke, partly to reduce the amount of water it carries, and mainly to remove any particles of grit or dirt that might separate the rubber from the glass. It also eliminates the danger of scratching the window.

High windows can often be cleaned by using terry towelling around a squeegee on an extension pole as the detergent applicator, and then using the squeegee in the normal way to clean. Extension poles up to 12 feet long can be handled with little practice.

WINDOW CLEANING IN NEW BUILDINGS

The problem is sometimes encountered of cleaning windows in new premises, or after extensive remodeling or alterations have been carried out. In most cases, the windows are left covered with patches of plaster, putty of various types, paint, and even cement or mortar. On the other hand, the paintwork around the windows will probably be new, and therefore slightly soft, so that any cleaning process has to be designed to remove heavy deposits from the glass without damaging the surrounding paint.

The best procedure is as follows. Cover the paintwork at the bottom of the window frame by placing cloth or newspaper over it, fastening the top edge of the shield to the glass with cellulose tape. The shield should be wide enough to cover the whole sill of the window frame. Using a painter's scraper or similar tool handled lightly, go over the window to remove as much as possible of the solid material, then sponge over with one of the proprietary liquid hard surface cleansers. This will loosen putty and paint, and they should now come off with an ordinary rubber squeegee. The window should then be rinsed with water, the paper or cloth shield removed from the sill, and the window squeegeed in the normal way, taking care not to press too hard on the paintwork at the edges.

An alternative to the proprietary cleanser (though not the same material) is a solution of diethanolamine at about one ounce per 1 ¼ pints of water. Diethanolamine is a mild alkali, chemically related to ammonia, but without the unpleasant fumes. It is quite a useful material for all hard surface cleansing, and does not need protective clothing or gloves.

# eight

# Carpets and Fittings

The care of carpets, furniture, furnishings and fittings may seem a simple matter compared with some of the more "technical" problems, because the work is similar to household maintenance. However, the maintenance manager will find it necessary to treat this section of his work very seriously, for two main reasons. First, just because the work is similar to housework, cleaners may assume that they know best how it should be carried out. They are often wrong, particularly about the least time-consuming way of doing the job, and consequently much labor cost may be expended on "trifling" household-type work. Second, the maintenance manager should consider where the best carpets, pieces of furniture, and so on are situated—under the constant eye of senior management. It is true, whether unfortunately or not, that the most efficient maintenance manager will find himself in trouble if the president's desk is dusty.

In this chapter, we shall consider the upkeep of carpets, upholstered and other furniture, and some of the more unusual materials that may be found in "prestige" parts of the building—marble, bronze, and the like.

## CARPETS

From one logical point of view, carpets could have been considered in the chapter on floorings, but the problems connected with their maintenance are quite different from those associated with hard flooring, and very similar to those found with other textile furnishings. It seems better, therefore, to give them a section of their own.

The idea of having a textile covering for the floor, with its consequent softness and warmth, is centuries old, and many types of construction have grown up in that time. The following brief descriptions will help to define the woven carpets, made by traditional methods.

1. *Aubusson tapestry:* Possibly the most beautiful carpets are made by this method. The hand-loomed variety may be distinguished by clear-cut ribs and small slits which are clearly discernible, together with a rough back and short ends of yarn visible on the back of the carpet. Machine-loomed Aubusson is more regular.

2. *Axminster:* A cut wool pile on a cotton or linen warp, and jute filling or weft (the pile is knotted to the weft).

3. *Brussels:* Rather like a Wilton carpet (below), but the loops made in the knotting are not cut, which makes the carpet feel rather less soft and silky than a Wilton.

4. *Oriental carpets:* In general each tuft is hand-knotted around the warp threads.

5. *Tapestry:* Constructed like a Brussels carpet, but printed, so the colors do not wear as well.

6. *Wilton:* A woolen or worsted pile (wool gives softness but tends to obscure the detail, while worsted is more erect and therefore stiffer, and shows the pattern better) closely woven with a separate warp pile for each color. The colors not in use are woven in under the others, adding to the strength and richness of the carpet.

Knotted or woven carpets are obviously out of the question for any but the most luxurious offices, and many of the cheaper methods produce carpets with inferior wearing properties. All this has, however, been altered by two developments of more recent years: the introduction of synthetic fibers, and the needlefelt method of making the pile. Needlefelt or needleloom carpets are made by a controlled process of ravelling the fibers.

In a typical process, woven hessian, nylon or jute, at the desired width for the carpet, is overlaid with several thicknesses of dyed jute, and then a number of layers of dyed nylon, rayon, or acrylic fiber to form the pile. This mattress, several inches deep, then passes through the needling machine, which contains hundreds of barbed needles moving up and down at high frequency. The barbs are arranged in the opposite direction to those of a fish hook or arrow, so that the needles tend to push threads down into the backing and systematically tangle them with one another. In general, the more needling, the better the resulting carpet; this is obviously governed by the speed at which the mattress is fed through the machine. Broken needles, which often occur, are removed by electromagnets, and any recalcitrant fragments are found by metal detectors and removed by hand. The back of the carpet is covered with a paste of vinyl or rubber latex, sometimes with foam rubber or plastic included to make a built-in carpet pad, and this is cooked to set it around the bottoms of the fibers. Finally, the top of the pile is trimmed level and the carpeting is ready for sale.

Many variations are possible using different types or mixtures of fibers for the pile, the backing, and the coating, and the use of hard-wearing materials such as polypropylene promises to give needlefelt carpeting a service life equal to that of knotted carpets, and able to stand up to the heaviest industrial use.

The great enemy of all carpets is grit. While grit may be merely unsightly on a concrete or plastic floor, and may dull linoleum and cork, it can literally cut a carpet to pieces. Grit sinks into the pile of carpets, and every step, because of the resilience of the carpeting, means that the threads in the pile in the underfoot area are being rubbed to and fro against the sharp edges of the gritty particles—an effect on the small scale like taking a stone axe to the carpet. Regular and thorough vacuuming of carpets is therefore essential not only for appearance, but also to lengthen the life of the floor covering.

Vacuuming, however, will only remove the easily removable grit. Grit which is stuck to the pile by grease, sticky food particles and so on, must also be removed, and here it is necessary to turn to wet-cleaning methods of removal.

Moisture is also an enemy of carpets. It swells fibers (even synthetic ones to some extent), it loosens the backing and tends to encourage mold growth unless dried off very thoroughly—a matter of some difficulty with an object like a carpet, that is laid flat on the floor. Commercial carpet cleaners operate in such a way as to minimize the amount of water used in cleaning, and to make sure that the drying is really adequate (I am speaking here, of course, of *competent* commercial carpet cleaning—I have seen a heavy industrial scrubber taken over a customer's carpet, followed by hosing with hot water and "hanging up to dry," a procedure calculated to shorten the life of the carpet by 20 per cent at least). It is not always convenient to have the carpet taken up for outside cleaners to operate, and in hotels, for instance, this may mean that the space is unusable for three or more days.

The alternative is to clean the carpet on the premises, and here the main problem is rinsing adequately and getting the carpet dry again. In fact it is impossible to rinse properly, so the type and method of application of the detergent must be modified to allow for this. Ordinary liquid detergents are not really suitable for carpet cleaning. Because all the detergent cannot be rinsed out, traces of detergent material will be left in the pile after drying. Most nonionic detergents in the concentrated form are liquids; most anionic detergents are waxy solids. The effect is that the carpet is left impregnated with sticky detergent which not only retains residual dirt but actually attracts more soiling from shoes. Additionally, the pile of the carpet loses its fluffiness and resilience because the fibers are stuck together.

The ideal method of cleaning carpets on the premises is to produce a foam from some variety of detergent that dries to a completely non-sticky powder. Such detergents are lithium lauryl sulfate, sodium lauryl sulfate, lithium lauryl ether sulfates, sodium lauryl sarcosinate, and several other types. The theoretical choice of products is very wide. Most of these materials are not very soluble in water, and indeed it might be said that their readiness to crystallize out of solution is a measure of their efficiency in drying out completely. To make them into suitable solutions for use, they usually need to have other materials added to them to increase their solubility. Alcohol is often used. The favorite concentration for sale is about 10 per cent of detergent in a mixture of alcohol and water; this is diluted to 1 per cent for use.

A typical shampooing operation is carried out as follows: The carpet is thoroughly vacuumed to remove as much surface dirt and loose grit as possible, then it is spread with a layer of foam made from the carpet shampoo as 1 per cent active detergent in warm water. For small areas a sponge or brush is satisfactory for application, but for large areas of carpeting a machine is better. A floor machine fitted with soft nylon brushes is effective. The aim should be to cover the carpet with foam, using the absolute minimum amount of solution to do this, so that the backing of the carpet is wetted as little as possible. The foam rapidly sinks into the carpet, and operators should be warned against the natural tendency to add more detergent to "build up" the foam again. As it sinks into the pile the foam will loosen and suspend dirt, and remove grease and sticky materials, and therefore lift the dirt free of the fibers. If the carpet is very dirty, as shown by the foam becoming brown or even black even before it sinks into the pile, the detergent can be picked up by wet suction and a further treatment given, but this should not be done unless it is really imperative.

For very large areas, the following procedure is appropriate. It makes use of a floor machine, suitable to the size of the carpet, and a wet suction machine.

1. Fill the tank of the scrubbing machine with warm water and the correct dilution of carpet shampoo.

2. The operators should position themselves at right angles to one another, then commence at the furthermost corner of the room from the door and work backwards to avoid walking on the wet carpet.

3. The drying unit should follow the scrubber and remove the shampoo foam immediately. It is important that moisture should not penetrate to the carpet backing.

4. After completing one strip of carpet, the brushes of the scrubber are lifted off the carpet and the machine is moved to the next strip, again starting at the top of the carpet and moving back. This procedure is followed until the entire carpet has been covered.

5. It is important that the carpet should not be walked on for at least one hour after shampooing.

When the carpet is dry (i.e. about two hours on a warm summer day, three to four hours at least in the winter, and sometimes as long as 12 hours; the detergent must be allowed to become entirely desiccated) it is thoroughly vacuumed again. This removes the mixture of dry detergent and dirt, and lifts the pile of the carpet to give it an entirely refreshed appearance.

Machines which combine the brushing action and wet suction are available from several manufacturers. A typical machine has two contra-rotating cylindrical brushes (four inches in diameter x 16 inches wide), supplied with foam by means of a shampoo tank feeding its solution through a blower. The foam so produced is about 90 per cent air and 10 percent solution, so the risk of overwetting is minimized even with careless handling. The foam is picked up by a squeegee and vacuum system similar to that in most suction dryers. There is a five gallon pick-up tank. The machine weighs 85 pounds and Figure 8.1 shows most of the details of the mechanism. The manufacturers claim that a carpet cleaned in this way can be dry again in one hour.

The choice of detergent materials is reasonably wide, and most large detergent manufacturers, and some machinery manufacturers, will provide a carpet shampoo, some with a germicide included. The buyer should always insist that the product contains an effective anti-corrosion agent. This is because it is often impossible to remove all heavy items of furniture from a room before shampooing, and metal casters or feet may be resting for hours on a carpet that is damp with shampoo. Unless the solution is properly inhibited, rust will develop and this will stain the carpet. An additional precaution, used by professional carpet cleaners, is to place small pieces of polythene or even waxed paper under each leg of heavy furniture.

It is possible to use "built" detergent powders for carpet shampooing, but they do not dry out as well as the specially-formulated materials,

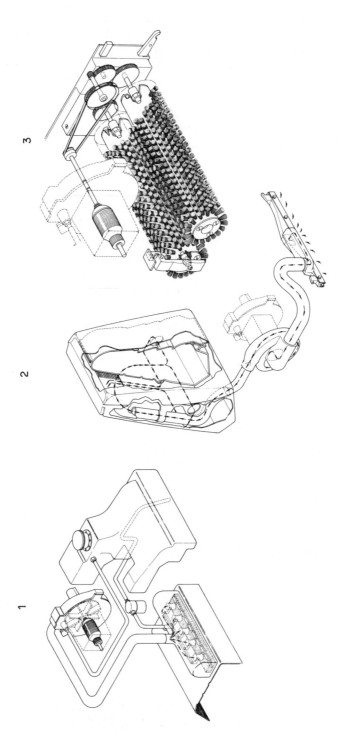

Figure 8.1

Carpematic machine. (1) Foam-producing mechanism. (2) Foam-removing mechanism. (3) Brush mechanism. (Acknowledgments to Protasil Ltd.)

and the alkalis which they contain may affect the color of the carpet. On balance, while such products may be cheaper than carpet shampoos, their use is a doubtful economy.

ANTI-STATIC TREATMENTS

One common problem with carpets, especially if they are laid over underfloor heating systems, is that they tend to generate static electricity as people move over them, and this electric charge spreads to the people themselves. This is particularly serious with nylon and acrylic fiber carpets. When the users of the room touch any grounded object, such as a light switch, telephone, or metal window frame, they receive a shock which can be painful and is always disconcerting. I have had personal experience of an office where a scientist was in the habit of pacing the room while thinking over problems in his work. After a particularly painful series of shocks, the telephone, lighting system, and even the lightning conductor system of the building were laboriously overhauled, until it was at last realized that the electricity was coming from a nylon carpet over underfloor heating, and the telephone, switches, and so on were merely acting as conductors.

Apart from annoyance to personnel, electrical apparatus can be affected by static charges generated from carpets, and again, if the real source is not suspected, much time may be wasted looking for faults in the apparatus itself. pH meters and any equipment of the tube voltmeter type tend to be affected in this way.

The cure is to make the carpet itself a conductor of electricity, and there are several proprietary dressings that can be used. Nearly all of them are based on quaternary ammonium compounds, and a very satisfactory result can be obtained with a 2 per cent solution of benzalkonium chloride lightly sprayed over the carpet. One spraying will last for a very long time, but the treatment must be renewed after shampooing the carpet, because not only will the anti-static agent be removed by washing, but quaternary ammonium compounds will be inactivated by the anionic detergents used for shampooing.

ANTI-STAIN TREATMENTS

Silicones can be used to protect a carpet against spilling, and proprietary dressings are available for this purpose. These cut down the water absorption of the fibers, and make them more resistant to spills such as coffee, beer, wine, mud, animal droppings and paint. They are thus very useful for caterers, schools, and hospitals. Spills that would normally spread and stain can usually be picked up with a cloth or sponge from a silicone-treated carpet. Such treatment is very desirable after carpet shampooing, as traces of detergent left in the carpet (even after careful vacuuming, there will be some traces) tend to increase the water absorption of the fabric by acting as wetting agents, and this means that spills can penetrate further into the carpet than they normally would.

The cleaning and maintenance of upholstered furniture, apart from routine dry vacuuming, presents the same problems as those involved in carpet care. The fabric must not be wetted too much, rinsing is virtually impossible, and drying is difficult.

## UPHOLSTERY

Fortunately the same "dry-foam" technique can be used as for carpets. The shampoo, at about 1 per cent active detergent concentration, is spread over the upholstery with a brush or sponge, so as to create as much foam as possible with the minimum amount of liquid. The furniture is then brushed vigorously with a soft-bristled brush, using a circular movement for looped-pile fabrics and a straight movement for cut-pile or velvet fabrics. This is followed ideally by suction drying, if a machine with an extension is available; in any case, the furniture is left to dry. Assistance from a radiator or even a hand hair dryer is useful at this stage. The surface is then thoroughly vacuumed to remove the mixture of dirt and dry detergent.

Such treatment, using lithium lauryl sulfate as the detergent, has been used successfully on the priceless antique furniture in the Victoria and Albert Museum, London, England, and most of the proprietary carpet shampoos sold by reputable detergent manufacturers will be found suitable for upholstery also. If the material seems particularly delicate or there is any reason to doubt the fastness of the fabric, a small test area can usually be found in an inconspicuous place (behind the seat of a chair, for instance) to try out the shampoo before applying it to the whole of the upholstery. As with carpets, the buyer should insist that a shampoo used for upholstery must have an effective corrosion inhibitor; otherwise furniture nails and other metal objects may produce rust marks on the fabric as it dries.

Alternatively, upholstery may be dry-cleaned using a suitable solvent: trichloroethylene or preferably tetrachloroethylene (perchloroethylene) is satisfactory for most fabrics. For spotting, a small quantity of the solvent should be spread on a pad of lint-free cloth and worked lightly from the center of the grease spot to the outside, carrying on the line until a point is reached where the solvent on the pad is almost exhausted and can hardly be seen to wet the upholstery fabric. Carry on like this, radially from the center, until the solvent has been spread regularly in all directions, and the outer points of the circle are scarcely distinguishable. This technique, known to the dry cleaner as "feathering out," is the only effective way to avoid marking the upholstery with rings. If solvent is poured straight onto a grease spot it spreads out in a circle, carrying the grease to its outside edge, and finally leaving a dark circle of grease which may be more unsightly than the original spot.

After the solvent has been spread out in this way, any excess is mopped up with lint-free cotton. The action of *gentle* heat from an electric iron over the cotton may assist in drying and finishing off evenly.

For really delicate fabrics, the fluorinated solvent Freon 113 (trifluorotrichloroethane, E.I. du Pont de Nemours) may be used for dry cleaning. It is extremely mild in its action, and does not appear to affect any normal type of fabric or dyestuff. However, it is several times more expensive than perchloroethylene.

In all cases, work of this kind with solvents must be carried out in a well-ventilated place, and operators should take care not to breathe the vapors directly. While the dangers of long-term liver damage, which used to be common with users of chlorinated solvents, are much less considerable with the three solvents mentioned above, there is the simple danger of narcosis; all solvents of this kind have a more or less anesthetic effect. Operators should not smoke during dry cleaning.

Dry cleaning cannot be recommended for large-scale use on upholstered furniture, as the solvents will also remove varnish and polish from woodwork; white spirit might be a possible exception to this, but suffers from the dangers of flammability. Aqueous shampooing is much safer from all points of view.

## LEATHER

Leather, as used for furniture, desk tops, decorative panels and other features in a building, is almost invariably what the tanner calls "light leather." All leather comes from the hides of animals. The easily-rotted keratin and globular proteins from the outside of the skin are removed by treatment with alkalis and enzymes ("liming") to leave a strong net of collagen, the main structural material of the skin. This collagen would itself rot if left to the action of bacteria, but it is tanned. This is a chemical modification which links the collagen molecules together and makes them less easily decomposed by bacteria and less easily penetrated by water.

Tough leathers, for the soles of shoes and similar purposes, are tanned at a fairly high temperature using vegetable tannins; these are "heavy leathers." Shoe uppers, furniture, and most other decorative leathers are tanned cold, usually with compounds of chromium or similar metals.

Leather is thus a network of fibers, and more like a textile than, say, a plastic sheet. It tends to absorb liquids in the same way that textiles do, and may give trouble with staining. The greatest danger to leather is damp heat; water at any temperature over moderately warm tends to convert the collagen to much softer proteins resembling gelatin, and irreversible damage takes place. The leather becomes shiny and brittle, usually darkens, and begins to flake away. Old leather, such as is found in antique furniture and bookbindings, may deteriorate in this way with alarming speed, so if leather gets wet, it should never, under any circumstances, be dried by artificial heating.

The best way to avoid penetration by water is to dress the leather with a good wax polish or with saddle soap. Light leathers are usually lubricated with an emulsion of oil ("fat liquoring") during manufacture, but it tends to lose its effectiveness after a time, and some sort of waxy material will give the leather new suppleness and also make it less easily wetted. Liquid waxes are quite suitable, but a saddle soap containing about 10 per cent soap and 30 per cent wax (carnauba, beeswax, or other hard waxes mixed with neatsfoot oil) will give a better result for furniture or automobile upholstery. Stains on leather are difficult to remove without damage to the material itself; ink and rust may be lightened with a jelly made from sodium citrate (2 ½ ounces to 1 pint of water) and enough cellulose wallpaper paste to give a suitable consistency to stop the solution from running. Ballpoint pen ink can be removed with alcohol, though it may be necessary to go over the area with wax polish, "feathered-out," to conceal the defatting effect of the spirit. Tar, rubber, fresh paint and similar materials can be removed with white spirit, but again the patch will need to be repolished to restore the leather to its pristine state.

## TELEPHONES

Modern standards of hygiene demand that the telephone, the target for so many bacteria as well as words, should be disinfected regularly. Even if telephones are not shared, the user may re-infect himself day after day from the mouthpiece, and the hard, non-absorbent surface, though it will not allow the growth of bacteria, can carry many spores. The best way to clean a telephone and render it reasonably sanitized is to wipe it with a solution of cationic germicide at about one per cent concentration, or one of the commercial mixtures of nonionic and cationic detergents sold as germicidal cleansers. Many telephone companies require the cleansing agent to pass their own tests for safety to the instruments. Mixtures containing alcohol or other solvents are not usually permitted, nor are products containing abrasives.

The alternative is to engage one of the companies who will clean and disinfect instruments weekly, and, of course, use approved materials.

## VENETIAN BLINDS

Slatted blinds, very popular with offices with a large window area, are a nuisance to clean. They present a great deal of surface area—a drop blind covering a window eight feet by six feet will have about 120 square feet of surface, counting both sides of the slats and the overlapping edges. The surfaces are difficult to get at because of the narrow spacing between the slats, and the blind presents no firm surface for the cleaner.

For on-the-premises cleaning, the best solution is a powerful vacuum cleaner fitted with a small brush head. Multiple brushes are available, but experience seems to show that these take so long to fit into the spaces that a single brush is equally efficient. Hand brushing and dusting is a very slow operation, and the parts of the blinds near the cords usually remain neglected.

For more thorough cleaning it is usually best, and quickest, to take the blinds down and wash them, using a large amount of agitation. Alkaline detergents should not be used, especially on aluminum slats, and the best method is either:

1. To wash the blind in a blend of nonionic and cationic detergent, at about 1/5 ounce per gallon of a 25 per cent active detergent product, or
2. To wash the blind in a solution of nonionic detergent, and follow this up with a rinse in dilute cationic detergent at about 1/10 ounce per gallon.

The purpose of the cationic detergent, in both methods, is to render the surface of the blinds less liable to pick up static electricity, which tends to attract dust.

Pitting of aluminum slats is caused by corrosion from the atmosphere, or it may be caused by unwise use of alkaline detergents in cleaning. It makes the slats much more liable to pick up dirt, and when the pitting has gone very far the blinds must be reslatted; from the point of view of cleaning, the sooner the better after pitting has started. The edges of the slats pit first, especially the edge facing the window, so a finger run along the outside of the slat may reveal pitting before it has gone very far.

## DECORATIVE FITTINGS

It is impossible to list all the materials used in decorative fittings, but a few general notes may be given for the commonest types of fitting.

### Marbles

Marble in the form of statuary or decorative architectural features should be cleaned only with liquid neutral detergents, preferably nonionic detergent solution at about 1/10 ounce per gallon of the 25 per cent material. Marble is very sensitive to acids, which rapidly etch it, and to a lesser extent to alkalis, which can penetrate microscopic gaps in it and cause cracking or flaking. Soap, soap powders and built detergent powders should be avoided. A coating or liquid wax polish or emulsion polish is the best protective treatment. Rust marks can sometimes be removed with a poultice of sodium citrate (1 ounce to 1/3 pint of water) mixed with whiting to a smooth paste, but this should not be left on for more than about 20 minutes.

### Brass and Bronze

Brass and bronze decorative features should be cleaned with metal polish and then lacquered, using a clear lacquer of the cellulose butyrate type. If green stains develop under the lacquer of a bronze object, strip off the old lacquer with a solvent paint stripper or trichloroethylene. The stains can be cleaned off with metal polish and the bronze relacquered.

### Clear Plastic and Epoxy Resins

Some display pieces are made either in polymethyl methacrylate ("Perspex") or epoxy resin. In both cases the main danger is scratching and crazing the surface, which will spoil the transparency of the plastic. Scouring powders and pastes should never be used on the plastics, and most solvents should not be allowed to contact them. Strong bleach solutions will damage Perspex, but not epoxy resins. For the removal of difficult soiling, nonionic detergent, alcohol, or white spirit may be used, with caution.

# nine

# Exteriors

The structure of a building, particularly if it is brick or concrete, looks so massive and permanent that it is difficult to think of it as ever changing. Unfortunately this is not true, by any means. Every building is undergoing constant attack by the elements—rain eroding as it runs down the surface, or setting up strains by absorption or freezing and thawing; soot and other dirt penetrating the surface; and, worst, acid in the atmosphere setting up chemical attack. Nearly all the fuels that are used for heating, in power stations and in vehicles, contain small quantities of sulfur or its compounds. When these fuels are burned, the sulfur is converted to the gas sulfur dioxide, and this slowly oxidizes in the atmosphere to sulfur trioxide, which combines with rain to make sulfuric acid. The proportions of sulfur in any given sample of fuel may be very small, but the total amount of fuel used in a modern industrial environment is so huge that the air over a large city contains literally tons of sulfuric acid. This situation is well summed up in the unemotional wording of the building textbooks: "soaking the stone for a few days in a 1 per cent solution of sulfuric and hydrochloric acids will show whether it will be durable in a city atmosphere."

## BRICKWORK

Well-made bricks are among the most resistant of masonry materials. They stand up well to the effects of rain and acid atmospheres. Unfortunately the brick itself is not the whole of the wall, for quite a large proportion is mortar. Mortar is very complex chemically, but it is not too great a simplification to say that it behaves, to the atmosphere,

*175*

like a very soft limestone. It is readily attacked by the acid in the air, and, being very porous, tends to soak up water, which dissolves out the lime from the mortar and may cause cracking in freezing weather. Also, in the thousands of individual bricks that make up a wall, there are sure to be some of lower quality, with cinders, iron oxide, cracks, and other weak points, so that the rain and acids can penetrate and cause cracking.

If the surface of the bricks is very dense, as in best quality facing brick, soot and dirt will not penetrate to any significant extent; but in lower quality bricks the surface itself provides innumerable small holes which gradually fill up with water and soiling matter. This can be removed from small areas of brickwork by the use of a solution of nonionic detergent of the nonylphenol condensate type, at about ¼ ounce per gallon, using ordinary bristle brushes to provide the mechanical action. Anionic detergents should not be used, either alone or in blends with nonionics, as the penetration of mortar by these materials, nearly all of which contain sulfates, may lead to erosion and cracking of the mortar. The nonionic detergent should not give excessive lather under these conditions, but if foam is causing a nuisance, the amount of detergent can be reduced. The cleansing power of the solution will of course be reduced in proportion.

When large areas of brickwork, for instance a whole building, are to be cleaned, the use of detergent in these amounts would be prohibitively expensive, and disposal of the detergent solution would also be a problem. The best answer in such cases is the use of water and brushes alone, with the water applied in the form of a very fine mist by means of special nozzles fitted to pressure hoses. Such treatment has the advantage that the amount of water used is relatively small, and therefore the arrangements for supply and disposal are easier. Because no detergents or other cleansers are used, the spray cannot do any damage if it should chance to fall on sidewalks or be swept by the wind past the protective screens and over passers-by.

While the scaffolding is still up for cleaning purposes, it is obviously the ideal time to apply a water-repellent treatment to reduce the penetration of water and other liquids into the brickwork, and, more important, the mortar. A silicone-based proofing treatment is ideal for this purpose, as it has the property of preventing the entry of liquid water without sealing in water vapor, so that moisture already in the masonry can escape without causing blistering or other attack on the water-repellent layer. Not all silicone treatments are suitable for use immediately after cleaning, but there are now on the market water-based emulsions of silicone oils which are quite safe at this time. Such treatment must of course wait until all repair or restoration work is complete; otherwise the proofing effect of the silicone oil is likely to interfere with the adhesion of the cement, mortar, or other building materials.

## STONEWORK

Building stones may be divided into three main groups: limestones, sandstones, and granite.

### Limestones

These consist mainly of calcium carbonate with small amounts of other materials. *Compact* limestones contain this carbonate mixed evenly with small amounts of clay or sand; granular or *oolitic* limestones consist of grains of calcium carbonate, often egg-shaped (hence the name oolitic), cemented together by sand and clay or finely divided calcium carbonate; *shelly* limestones consist of small shells cemented in a similar way; while *magnesian* limestones contain more than 15 per cent of magnesia in addition to calcium carbonate. *Dolomites* are a particularly hard form of magnesian limestone containing equal proportions of calcium and magnesium carbonates. Portland stone is a good example of building limestone. *Marble* can also be considered as a form of limestone, as it is chemically similar, but has been crystallized by heat and pressure.

All limestones are attacked by acids very readily and are therefore susceptible to the action of the acids in the atmosphere, the sulfuric acid changing calcium carbonate to the much more soluble calcium sulfate. They also take up soot readily, and can turn from white to all shades of brown to black.

Most limestones have the property of being "self-cleansing" to some extent. The soot covering them rests on the outer layer of calcium carbonate, and as this is converted to calcium sulfate by the acid atmosphere, or more slowly into calcium bicarbonate by the carbon dioxide of the atmosphere, the outer layer slowly dissolves in rain water and carries away the soot with it. This can make the appearance of a building worse, because the features exposed to rain, or the upper parts generally, remain cleaner than sheltered or low-lying parts, and the contrast between the two shows up the grime even more than a uniform coating of soot would do.

The best method of cleaning is to imitate the action of rain in a controlled way, i.e. to spray the stonework with water, using a jet which produces a fine spray. After thorough wetting of the stone, so as to loosen the deposits to some extent, dirt can be removed by high-pressure water sprays, brushing, or abrasion, according to the situation and depth of the soiling. Experiments have been carried out to see whether the addition of detergents, wetting agents, alkalis, or other materials added to the cleaning water would accelerate the cleaning process, but it has been shown that such additions do not have any useful effect at all, while of course adding immensely to the cost of the operation and the difficulties in disposing of the effluent.

Cleaning of limestone sometimes causes creamy-yellow stains on the surface; this seems to be due to colored materials, particularly iron salts, being dissolved by the water and brought to the surface. The iron could presumably be removed by treatment with sulfamic acid or a similar iron-dissolving agent, but this would mean serious etching of the limestone itself. Alternatively, one of the salts of ethylene diamine tetra-acetic acid (EDTA) specially intended for the removal of iron could be used, but the writer has no knowledge of such a process being tried, probably because of the cost.

An alternative treatment of limestone is sand-blasting under controlled conditions. This requires the services of skilled personnel, as the damage done by inexpert blasting is obviously almost irreparable, if details or carvings are affected. Sand blasting has the advantage that it cannot bring yellow stains to the surface, and it cannot affect iron cramps and dowels used to tie the stones in some older buildings, which might otherwise be encourage to rust by the soaking of the stone with water. The choice of water or sand-blasting will depend on several factors, including the size of the building, the accessibility, nearness to highways and sidewalks, and the amount of detail in the stone.

### Sandstone

This is composed of grains of sand (silica) held together by a cementing substance, which may be finely divided silica, alumina, calcium carbonate, or iron oxide. Those bound with silica are the most durable, those bound with iron oxide the least. If iron pyrites (iron sulfide) is present in the stone, it is certain to split or otherwise break up on weathering.

Siliceous sandstones are not much affected by the sulfuric acid in the atmosphere, but they tend to pick up soot readily in towns. This soot deposit is often very adherent, and the only reliable method for removal is dissolving away a small amount of the silica surface itself, using carefully controlled application of hydrofluoric acid. This acid dissolves silica to form hydrofluorosilic acid, and the layer of soot comes away with the silica. Hydrofluoric acid is a very dangerous chemical to use, being corrosive to almost all materials, including the skins and eyes of operators. Its use is only suitable for specially trained personnel with complete protective clothing and adequate shielding of the surrounding area.

A safer method of cleaning sandstone is to blast it with sand, carborundum, or, for buildings with fine detail, softer abrasives, such as copper slag and similar by-products of the metal industry.

## Granite

Granite is a volcanic rock composed mainly of quartz, feldspar, and mica, and it is extremely hard and impervious. Fortunately soot and dirt cannot penetrate very far into the stone, and the nebulous spray process that is suitable for limestone and brickwork is also suitable for granite. Alternatively, blasting can be used; sand or shot are suitable as the stone is so hard, but for delicate work softer abrasives may be used.

The cleaning of exterior stonework, except for small areas close to the ground, is almost exclusively a matter for contract companies with specialized personnel. The work needs complicated scaffolding, and the operators need not only to work high, but to support heavy brushing machines, high-pressure hoses, blasting equipment, and other hazardous machinery. The falling material, whether water, abrasive, or chemical solutions, must be disposed of without any possible nuisance to the general public or workpeople passing underneath, and the supply and disposal of large volumes of water for spraying may require special arrangements to be made with the water authorities. The major part of the cost of cleaning a large building is not, in fact, applying the cleaning agent to the surface, but making the arrangements to get it there.

## CONCRETE

Surfaces of concrete buildings may be cleaned in similar ways to those used for limestone. For small areas and the removal of local stains, the surface may be cleaned by the application of a solution containing about 1/10 ounce nonionic detergent (nonylphenol condensate at 25 per cent active detergent) and 2 ounces of sodium carbonate per gallon of water, brushed on and then scrubbed. Stains can be removed by following the general methods recommended for concrete floors in Chapter Six, using "poultice" methods to keep the active materials in contact with the wall.

## ALUMINUM

Anodized aluminum is used widely for the exteriors of buildings in factories and other commercial buildings, and it can form a very attractive and hygienic surface. For best results, the surface should never be treated with abrasive substances, as these will tend to spoil the anodized finish. Aluminum protects itself in the normal way by building up a layer of white aluminum oxide, which can become rough and scaly in appearance, although its protective powers remain the same. The anodizing process gives a controlled production of the oxide in a form that does not look as white and rough as the "natural" formation, yet gives the same protection. If a portion of the anodized finish is removed by abrasives, however, a patch of ordinary white oxide will form, standing out from the smooth finish of the rest of the surface.

The best treatment for exterior anodized aluminum, or even mill-finished aluminum, is to clean every three months with a solution of 1/5 ounce of nonionic detergent (nonylphenol condensate at 25 per cent active detergent) per gallon of hot water, using nylon bristle brushes if necessary to remove hard deposits. The ideal treatment, if the surface is not too large to make this economic, is then to apply a very thin coat of an acrylate emulsion polish, by mopping on from a dilute solution with a cellulose sponge mop or similar applicator, or to spray the solution on thinly. Such treatment gives a very fine finish to aluminum, increases the gloss, and makes the surface more resistant to dirt.

If the surface has been neglected or for any other reason there is a heavy deposit of dirt, a solvent/detergent mixture can be used for cleaning. This can either be one of the proprietary products of this type, or a mixture made up for the occasion with 1 ounce of nonionic detergent (at 25 per cent active detergent) and 1 ounce of white spirit per gallon of water. The emulsion so formed will not be stable, but the mixture will serve if agitated from time to time.

If the surface of aluminum has been allowed to accumulate loose oxide, the best treatment is to scrub it with nylon pads on a lightweight floor machine or one of the special wall washing machines, using a solution of *soap* as the cleansing agent. The soap may be made up in many ways; 2-3 ounces of domestic soap flakes or 1/5 ounce of liquid soap per gallon of water will make a suitable solution. The object of the soap is not only to assist in the cleansing of the aluminum surface, but also to coat it with a layer of aluminum soap which will prevent further oxide build-up. Aluminum oxide is difficult to remove from the surface of the metal, and as soon as it is removed, a new surface of oxide forms on exposure to air. Use of a soap solution allows the fresh aluminum surface to react with the soap before the air has a chance to get at it.

In cleaning exterior aluminum surfaces, it is as well to avoid treatment of these in the direct sun, as they become very hot, and the detergent or soap solution will dry in streaks before it is possible to rinse off. Probably because of reaction between the metal and the soap or detergent, these streaks are very permanent and cannot be removed without abrasion.

## FENCING AND WALLS

The maintenance manager should not forget that the exterior of building will usually also include boundary walls and fences, and other built-up items that do not form part of the main mass of the building. Walls and similar structures should be treated according to their materials of construction—concrete, brick, or other material.

Wire fences and similar metal boundary markers do not usually require much maintenance, but weeds growing around them can cause rapid rusting and other corrosion. Weeds tend to prevent moisture from draining away from the fence and cut down evaporation, so that the fence stays moist for very much longer than it would if free of plant life. The best treatment is to use a general weed killer such as sodium chlorate crystals scattered around the fence; this will rapidly cause the weeds to dry up, and they can easily be removed. The same treatment can be applied to plants such as moss and lichen growing on the footings of buildings or masonry walls. Such growths encourage dampness and may cause cracking.

# ten

# Kitchens

Kitchens and similar food preparation areas are a great responsibility for the maintenance manager, for two reasons. They are, by the nature of the work carried out, more likely to become dirty and greasy than any other area of the building, and the consequences of any neglect are likely to be serious—the spread of bacteria and molds, food poisoning, wastage of food by spoilage, and the encouragement of vermin, which bring with themselves more health hazards. Food preparation and serving are also costly operations and deserve separate study in every aspect, including the most efficient methods of cleaning and maintaining kitchen fittings and cooking ware, and dishwashing.

The rapid growth of the use of vending machines, for food and drink, is a natural consequence of the high labor cost of food serving. This development has brought in its train new problems of cleaning and maintenance, and new health hazards. These also will be considered in this chapter.

## KITCHEN PREMISES

It is impossible to maintain adequate hygiene in a kitchen unless the area itself is constructed and finished to assist in the work of cleaning. Floors and walls should be smooth and impervious with all angles coved, including the angles between the floor and walls, the junctions of the walls, and between the walls and ceiling. When the walls are not tiled, it is necessary to plaster with a very hard and smooth coating, and preferable to cover this with gloss paint or a smooth plastic which can be washed regularly without losing its smooth surface. Whitewash, calcimine, and similar rough coatings are quite unsuitable. The floor should be continuous also. Concrete is not very easy to keep clean, and asphalt tends to harbor dirt and grease in scratches, but terrazzo, quarries or latex cement are satisfactory. Probably the best flooring for a kitchen is a concrete subfloor covered with a generous coating of polyurethane resin: this is continuous, easy to keep clean, attractive in appearance, and has a good non-slip surface, even when wet or greasy. Floorboards of ordinary softwood are quite unsuitable. They shrink, resulting in open joints, and in these gaps food waste and grease can collect. Bacteria multiply in the pores of the wood, and vermin such as roaches can live in the subfloor cavity and come up through the cracks between the boards.

Sinks should be of stainless steel or porcelain, and so should drainboards. Edging pieces of wood should be avoided, as they often become miniature cesspools in which food residues collect and bacteria and roaches breed.

It is important that drainage pipes should be trapped as close as possible to the sinks, and discharge through the wall into a suitable drain. Waste water from washing up sinks should discharge through a proper grease-trap, and waste water from potato peeling machines and similar sources of solid residues should have a strainer or silt trap before the water reaches the drainage system. It is not good practice to allow the drainage of water into internal drains, because too often the cleaning of these is neglected and they become serious sources of infection. Only when they actually block or begin to smell do people take the trouble to clear them out. Drains and grease traps should be cleaned at least twice a week, and silt traps after each use of the machine which they serve.

Preparation tables should always be movable, and if they are set against a wall no backboards should be used. It is far better for a small amount of food to fall onto the floor from the back of a preparation table (where it will be seen and cleaned up) than for scraps to collect behind a backing board. The working tops of tables should be coated with a continuous laminated plastic surface, except for butcher's cutting, which can be carried out on a hardwood block such as sycamore or similar close-grained wood.

A half-channel drain should surround all cooking equipment, covered by a grating, and the floor should have gentle slope to this channel. This facilitates the emptying of boilers, steamers and similar equipment, and encourages the staff to wash the floors with plenty of water. Daily cleaning of the channel and drain is essential.

A wash basin in the kitchen with hot and cold water, soap, nail brush and towels or a hand dryer is essential. Personnel should be told, and continually reminded, that a very high standard of hygiene is necessary for food workers, and such practices as ear, nose and head scratching, licking of the fingers and many worse habits are all real hazards to the health of people to whom they supply food. A notice must be displayed in the toilet reminding staff to wash their hands after using it. Clothing and footwear must not be left in the food preparation area.

Refuse and waste food must be removed from the kitchen at once and placed in metal or plastic garbage containers fitted with tight lids. If these can be stored under cover and in an area safe from dogs, cats, and children, it is better. A trellis or other open type of fence will give reasonable security without preventing ventilation.

## REFRIGERATORS

Maintenance of the refrigerator is a very important part of kitchen management. The container should not be crowded with foodstuffs, and strict priority should be given to foodstuffs such as cooked meats, pates, and soups. Canned food, which is often found in refrigerators, does not need to be protected in this way at all. Cheese, butter, fats, and oils need far less protection than cooked meat.

Meat cooked on the day prior to serving should be cooled quickly in a cooling area prior to placing it in the refrigerator. On no account place hot meat in the refrigerator to cool it: this will overload the cooling system and cause condensation, and the meat itself may become offensive when taken out again. Hot meat and similar dishes should not be left in the kitchen overnight.

Rapid cooling is essential because the dangerous food poisoning organism *Clostridium welchii* can grow rapidly in warm meat, and if it passes into the spore form, can resist quite high temperatures of cooking. "Cook and eat the same day" is the best way to avoid *Clostridium welchii* infection, but if this is not feasible, then cool the meat as quickly as possible. The use of small fans and ample ventilation in the food storeroom will all assist.

## PERSONNEL HYGIENE

Apart from the hand washing mentioned before, personnel must be provided with first aid equipment to enable them to dress and cover cuts and abrasions as soon as possible. Bandaging is not satisfactory, especially for hands or fingers, as the bandage soon becomes saturated and infected material can still be passed onto food. Waterproof dressings are therefore necessary.

Food workers suffering from infected wounds, cuts, boils, or any staphylococcal infection should not be allowed to handle food, equipment, or anything else in the kitchen. Persons suffering from diarrhea should similarly be barred from the kitchen, and personnel with any intestinal disorder bad enough to keep them from work should not be allowed in the kitchen again until they have a doctor's clearance. Smoking in the food preparation area ought to be prohibited.

The provision of suitable premises and regulations for the preparation of food is not just a matter of staying within the law. The upkeep of a kitchen in a clean state is an expensive business under the best conditions, and if the premises are not well adapted to be kept clean, or if the employees have dirty habits, the costs of day-to-day running become much higher than they should be. The capital outlay required to bring premises into a hygienic state can be recouped in a very short time by savings in running costs, less wastage and spoilage of food, smaller turnover of personnel and more efficient operation generally.

## KITCHEN EQUIPMENT

### POTS AND PANS

In the cleaning of pans, saucepans and similar ware, this advice is still the best that can be offered: "A saucepan filled with water begins to clean itself." Starches and proteins both tend to become harder and more insoluble through irreversible reactions as they lose water, the starches becoming more like gums, and the proteins becoming "denatured" (which is a rather vague word denoting a loss of solubility and other properties of "living" protein) and also very adherent to surfaces. If a saucepan is allowed to dry with starch or protein residues on it, cleaning is therefore very much more difficult than it would be if the pan had been filled with cold water as soon as possible after use.

Many detergent suppliers and managers of kitchens recommend the use of alkaline detergents for pot washing, and some of the products on the market contain quite large proportions of sodium carbonate or metasilicate. While alkali undoubtedly speeds up the removal of starch, it causes difficulties to the person actually carrying out the washing. He or she must use rubber gloves. In addition, alkaline detergents are not suitable for aluminum ware, which can be seriously corroded. A neutral liquid detergent combined with a nylon abrasive pad will normally remove residues just as fast as alkali, and with much more safety to the ware and the operators.

Where material has become burnt onto a vessel, the best treatment is to add a little sodium hypochlorite to the water used to soak the vessel, say 1/5 ounce (of the 10 per cent hypochlorite) to the gallon. If this does not remove all the carbonized material, make up a fresh solution of hypochlorite at about ½ ounce to the gallon, and bring this to the boil in the vessel to be cleaned. There may be faint darkening of aluminum by this treatment, but this will soon clear off with a nylon pad. Hypochlorite attacks all organic material, and therefore can attack heavy carbonized material, while alkali can only clean by decomposing the fat in the residues. If saucepans are being cleaned in this way, do not put nylon pads in the hypochlorite solution; it will attack the nylon and shorten the life of the pads drastically.

Some workers favor soap-filled steel wool pads for cleaning pots and pans. The soap tends to give a fine finish to aluminum and stainless steel particularly, possibly by forming a microscopic layer of insoluble metallic soap on the surface of the metal, but in general this treatment leaves a deposit of rather dirty soap and metal strands in the vessel which is difficult to wash out thoroughly.

SURFACES

The surfaces of all preparation tables, cabinets and similar parts of the kitchen can be a major factor in the spread of bacteria, with the consequent risk of disease. All surfaces should be cleaned with an effective germicide before and after use every day.

Phenolic compounds are not suitable for kitchen use because of their strong characteristic smell, which can be accompanied by an unpleasant taste at surprisingly low concentrations. One of the best general-purpose kitchen germicides is sodium hypochlorite. It is very powerful, destroys bacteria, molds, and yeasts, and has the advantage that after use it is decomposed into common salt, and can therefore leave no taint or smell. An excellent germicidal cleanser can be made by mixing 1/10 ounce of 10 per cent hypochlorite with 1/10 ounce of 25 per cent nonionic detergent per gallon of water. This should be used freely over all surfaces, particularly if wooden surfaces are used; wood, being more porous than plastic or metal, has many more crevices for organisms to shelter in. Alternatively, one of the proprietary mixtures of nonionic and cationic germicide may be used. Whichever is selected, it is important that a proper sequence of cleaning is laid down and adhered to. The casual wipe may impart false confidence that the premises are "clean," while bacteria are multiplying rapidly on some neglected piece of equipment.

Kitchen employees are usually hurried people, and are inclined to forget cleaning procedures unless it is made easy for them to remember. One or two simple precautions which can make a tremendous difference to the hygienic condition of a kitchen are as follows:

1. Always provide a plentiful supply of cleaning cloths and sponges, and insure that a simple marking (color, for instance) distinguishes those to be used on equipment and surfaces from those to be used on floors and walls.
2. Make sure that a plentiful supply of germicidal detergent is always available. The best method is to install a tap proportioner (see Chapter Five for details of these) so that it becomes automatic to add both detergent and germicide to cleaning water.
3. Do not permit cleaning cloths and sponges to be left about in the kitchen, but provide a suitable large vessel in which they can be kept in a germicidal solution.
4. Remind personnel, management, and the company accountant that a small increase in the usage of detergent and germicide will not cost as much as one case of food poisoning traced to the kitchen.

## FRYING EQUIPMENT

Deep fryers and other equipment containing frying fat or oil need special attention. Frying pans that are heavily carbonized will release small particles of carbon that settle on the food as black spots, and fat adhering to the carbon deposits is likely to become rancid very much faster than usual, and may spoil the whole batch of frying medium. Rancidity in fats and oils is caused by the formation of fatty acids, and high temperatures accelerate the process, so any burned regions set up rancidity very quickly.

Deep fryers should be drained of fat daily, the frying medium strained and residues of food and fat wiped out of the pan with a solution of 1/10 ounce sodium hypochlorite (10 per cent available chlorine) and 1/10 ounce nonionic detergent (25 per cent active) in a gallon of very hot water. The frying baskets and strainers must be cleaned as thoroughly as the pan itself. If despite this treatment there is any remaining baked-on carbon, fill the vessel with the cleaning mixture above and bring it to the boil. For slight carbonizing a lower concentration of hypochlorite and detergent may be sufficient. Then drain and rinse very thoroughly with hot water. Care should be taken in all cleaning operations on deep fryers not to damage the thermostat stem, which usually projects into the pan, and not to spill cleaning solution into gas flues or other pipework.

The same cleaning solution is useful for griddles, call-order installations, and similar equipment where large-scale frying or grilling takes place.

SINKS AND DRAINBOARDS

The same mixture can be used for cleaning and disinfecting sinks and drainboards, and has the advantage that it will remove stains from sinks, and help to destroy any food particles in traps and pipework.

## DISHWASHING

The ideal dishwashing method would remove all traces of food, lipstick and other soiling from dishes, glassware, and cutlery, sterilize the articles at the same time, and leave them bright, clean, sterile, and dry. In particular it would not leave any hazy water-spotting or streaks on glassware, it would not corrode, tarnish, or discolor cutlery (whether steel, stainless, cupro-nickel or silver), it would remove tannin stains from coffee and tea cups and saucers, lipstick from cups and forks, and dried-up egg, tomato ketchup, and similar residues from plates. It would also be cheap enough for use in the largest establishment with the greatest number of servings.

Such a method has not been found yet, but for every quality except the last, the nearest to ideal is hand dishwashing in soft water with a good detergent and a sterilizing sink. The difficulty is the matter of cost. Hand dishwashing is slow, and if it is done properly it is even slower than usual, and therefore expensive. An examination of the ideal method is none the less useful if only to underline some of the weaknesses of practical dishwashing methods.

The dishwashing sink should contain water as hot as the hands can bear it, with about 1/5 ounce per gallon of a germicidal detergent, preferably a mixture of nonionic and cationic detergent. Chlorinated materials could be used as the germicide, but they tend to discolor cutlery, and the odor of chlorine, particularly in greasy water, is sometimes unpleasant for the employees. The cationic germicides are virtually odor-free, and can leave no taint on dishes or cutlery. All parts of each article should be washed, with special attention to the handles, bases, and handle joints of cups, the handles of knives and forks as well as their blades and prongs, and the backs of plates as well as the fronts (readers who think that such details are superfluous should study a professional dishwasher at work). After washing, the articles should be rinsed briefly in clean hot water, and then immersed for at least one minute in water in a sterilizing sink at a temperature of 180° F (82° C) or higher, and finally taken out and allowed to dry without rubbing with a cloth. In practice, if a dishwasher observes all these details conscientiously, the output is about

600 pieces per hour or less. If the food happens to be difficult to remove (eggs and baked beans in tomato ketchup produce two of the dishwasher's bugbears), the rate may be much slower.

Even supposing that this ideal sequence has been learned, details soon begin to deteriorate. The sterilizing sink may be kept to temperature but the time of immersion may be far short of one minute, the period necessary for sterilization. Operators asked to assess the passage of one minute of time give such variable answers that it is impossible to believe that their use of the sterilizing sink is any more accurate. The use of a germicide in the detergent sink helps to minimize the ill-effects of carelessness, but the detergent itself has to be kept up to strength. Soon, unless supervision is close, the standard of mechanical cleansing is lowered, and the more difficult parts of the articles are not given the attention they need. In fact, while conscientious hand dishwashing can give the best results, too often it degenerates into the worst kind of unhygienic mess. This and the productivity factor explain the overwhelming preference for dishwashing machines in all branches of industry.

## JET MACHINES

If the required throughput of washed dishes and cutlery exceeds about 2,000 mixed pieces per hour (this corresponds roughly to about 200 meals per hour for a main meal service, or correspondingly more snacks or coffees) hand dishwashing becomes definitely uneconomic. It becomes too costly to pick up each article separately and wash it; the mechanical movement of the work has somehow to be automated. The jet dishwashing machine makes use of the mechanical energy of a rapid spray of detergent solution to clean soiling from the surface of the plates and cutlery, rather than following the hand method by immersing the work in detergent solution and applying the mechanical energy with a mop or brush.

In jet machines, the work is loaded into wire or plastic trays, which are designed to hold plates and so on at the right angle for maximum bombardment from the jets of detergent solution in the machine. Plates and saucers are placed with their concave side facing slightly upwards, cups upside-down so that the detergent solution will run out of them after they leave the machine. Cutlery is placed in wire baskets of a finer mesh, usually with a wire cover to hold the articles down, as the force of the jets can throw the light pieces of cutlery out of the basket altogether.

In smaller machines, these racks or trays are pushed into the machine by hand, and the jets allowed to impinge on them. Some machines generate most of the force of the jets by centrifugal force, but this is restricted to the very smallest. Most have a pump to provide the pressure. After washing with a detergent solution the work is rinsed with a fine but forcible jet of clean hot water, and then the tray is pulled out of the machine and another one pushed in. In these small machines, the main saving of time, compared with the ordinary household dishwashing machine, is in having several trays that can be used in the same machine. The housewife user arranges the work in her machine, sets the machine to wash, and then unloads the machine. The machine is thus only running for the wash, but occupied for all three operations, and often loading and unloading takes longer than the actual wash. In the industrial machine the trays can be loaded and unloaded away from the machine itself, and thus work can go on while the machine is washing other tray loads.

In larger machines the work of pushing trays into and out of the machine is largely mechanized by providing a mechanical conveyer inside the machine to carry the trays along. Figure 10.1 shows a diagrammatic view of a machine of this type. The baskets or trays are loaded with dishes, glassware, and cutlery in the normal way and placed on a table on the "inward" side of the machine; this table has a slight slope toward the machine so that spilled water and other liquids drain that way. The trays are then pushed gently by the operator until the wire or slats on the trays engage with the teeth of the conveyer, which can be a reciprocating driving arm or a roller chain conveyer. These devices keep the trays moving slowly through the machine at a rate calculated by the manufacturers to give adequate cleansing.

The trays pass first through a region with upper and lower jets of detergent solution at about 140° F (60° C), generated by pumping solution out of a central tank, through the pipework and jets, over the dishes and thence back to the detergent tank. Strainers in the bottom of the spraying area, placed over the detergent tank, prevent large pieces of bone, gristle, etc., from getting into the pumping mechanism or blocking the jets. The trays then enter a rinsing area, where upper and lower jets of clean water at about 180° F (82° C) wash the remaining detergent solution off them. In some machines this region is separate from the detergent region, but in most medium-sized machines the rinse water is disposed of by drainage into the detergent tank. To save overdiluting the detergent with too much rinse water, the rinse jets only come on when a tray is actually passing through; the control for this action is usually a pair of metal levers which are pushed back against the side of the machine by the passage of the tray, and thence open valves in the rinse line. Pressure switches similarly operated by the trays may be used. The trays after rinsing leave the machine and are pushed by the conveyer onto a slightly sloping table for unloading.

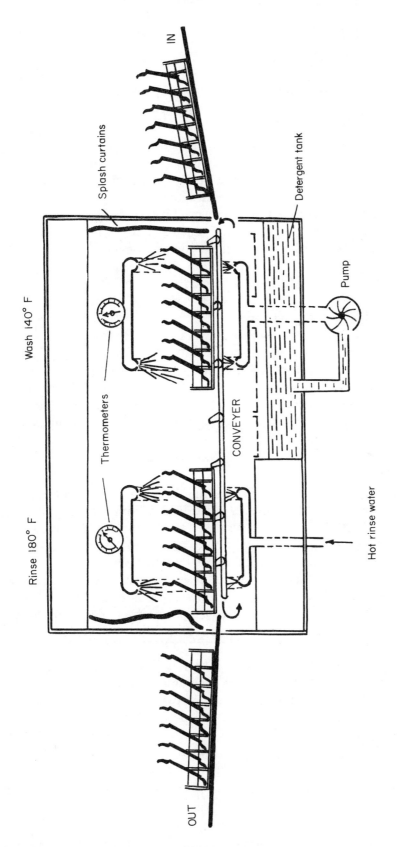

Figure 10.1

Typical conveyer dishwashing machine.

In the very largest machines, suitable for use in restaurants, drive-ins, and the like, with a very rapid turnover of customers, trays are dispensed with altogether and the conveyer consists of a continuous chain of pockets into which dirty items can be placed while the conveyer is moving, or a similar arrangement of steel pegs at the right angle to hold them. These "flight" type machines usually have separate detergent and rinse tanks, and the rinse is operated continuously.

To facilitate cleaning in all these machines, it is usual to make the jets (especially the detergent jets) fairly easy to remove for the elimination of scale, dirt, or any solid food which has somehow managed to escape the strainers. These strainers themselves are usually made up as detachable perforated trays fitting into the machine quite loosely, so that they can be removed after every period of use of the machine and emptied. This is essential if the machine is to work efficiently. Machines may be electrically, gas, or steam heated, and most of them have thermostats on the detergent and rinse lines with the ideal temperatures set.

The mode of action of jet machines is so far different from that in hand dishwashing that several specialized points of design and maintenance must be considered. Failure to take these into account may result in very poor quality work from an expensive machine, so they will be considered in some detail.

### Temperature

The temperature in hand dishwashing is limited by the tolerance of the human hand, and this imposes a practical maximum temperature of about 140° F (60° C). It might be supposed that in the machine, the higher temperatures which are possible would speed up the action of dirt removal, but it is found in practice that temperatures much over 140° F (60° C) tend to make some food residues more difficult to remove. Proteins such as egg and meat remains are set by heating, and may do so before the detergent has a chance to penetrate under them if the temperature is too high. The wash tank is therefore kept at about 140° F (60° C).

The rinse temperature 180° F (82° C) is designed to perform two functions. First, it sterilizes the work coming from the detergent jets, and second, it makes the dishes and glasses, in particular, hot enough to dry themselves by evaporation, thus avoiding the trouble and risk of bacterial contamination introduced by drying cloths. Any temperature above 180° F (80° C) would be satisfactory, but it is usually rather difficult to maintain the rinse much above this level because of the heat losses from the machine. A minor point is that a very hot rinse tends to fill the kitchen with steam unless the ventilation is good, but the main point is obviously the fuel cost.

### Re-Use of Detergent

It will be seen from Figure 10.1 that the detergent solution is recirculated time and time again during the operation of the machine, and therefore after the first few trays of work have gone through, fat and other soiling is also circulating. Large pieces of food are strained out, but it is still possible to find, in a large and busy kitchen, a liquid resembling soup rather than detergent solution circulating in the dishwashing machine at the end of a hectic lunch hour. In machines where the rinse-water drains back into the detergent tank, the detergent is steadily diluted with clean water, the volume being kept constant with a weir drainage device which helps to wash some of the soiling down the drain, but also diminishes the amount of detergent material in the wash liquid. It is necessary, therefore, to lay down detailed instructions for "topping-up" the detergent, and for changing the detergent solution entirely, at convenient slack times during the day. At the end of any dishwashing period the detergent should be discarded completely, and any food debris, stray cutlery, etc. removed from the strainers.

### Prewashing

Every particle of food debris left on the plates finds its way into the detergent solution, and therefore contributes towards an unsatisfactory result. If the type of food served is likely to result in residues—thick soups, sauces, and the like—a prewashing jet of water should be placed before the entry to the machine. The same applies to cups of coffee and other beverages, but if the cups are turned upside down before entering the machine the residues will be discarded automatically. The prewash water should be at about 120° F (49° C). For small installations a piece of flexible pipe fixed to a warm water tap is sufficient, while large machines are often provided with a prewash stage as part of the equipment.

### Detergents

Because all the mechanical action in a jet-type dishwasher proceeds from the force of the jets themselves, the agitation at the surface of a plate is tremendous, and a normal hand dishwashing type of detergent would be converted to a mass of foam in seconds. This is undesirable for two reasons: one is that the volume of foam can be embarrassing, with solid masses of foam being forced out of the machine, and, more important, the mechanical action of the jets is obstructed by the foam on the surface of the dishes. This effect is known as "fobbing." A detergent for jet-type machines must therefore have very low foaming power, and most of the conventional materials are ruled out.

Fortunately, the type of grease mainly encountered in dishwashing is animal or vegetable fat, and this is readily attacked by alkalis. The foundation of a successful machine dishwashing detergent is a mixture of alkalis: usually sodium carbonate, which is cheap; sodium metasilicate, which is more expensive but a more effective alkali; and trisodium phosphate, which is more expensive still, but invaluable for decomposing traces of protein material left on plates, as well as having the normal alkali effect on fats. In soft water such a mixture, with a very small amount of low-foaming wetting agent (there are several nonionics suitable for this, to be mixed with the alkalis at about 1/4-1/2 per cent), properly mixed into a dry non-caking powder, will give excellent results. It may be necessary to have a small amount of chlorinating agent to bleach cups, but this addition may not be so necessary in soft water. Too much chlorinating agent can cause tarnishing of cutlery, so it is best to keep the level of chlorine at about 30 p.p.m. in the detergent tank. If the powder is to be used as 1/2 ounce per gallon in the tank, for instance, the level of available chlorine in the powder should be about 0.8 per cent.

Unfortunately, when such a powder is used in hard water, the results are very poor. This is because all the alkalis react with calcium and magnesium salts in hard water to produce insoluble hydroxides (lime and magnesia, to use the common names), and these settle all over the dishes and glassware as a white film, with streaks and spots where drops of washing water have dried on the articles. As the hydroxides are insoluble, rinsing makes no great improvement. The only solution is to soften the water.

Water softening can be carried out in the machine by the addition of such materials as sodium sesquicarbonate, but the results will not be much better than with the alkaline powders themselves, because again insoluble material will be precipitated. The only effective softeners in the tank are the complex phosphates, sodium hexametaphosphate and sodium tripoly-phosphate. Sodium pyrophosphate can also be used, but has no advantage over the other two materials. The hexametaphosphate is readily available on the market and can be added by the machine operator, but it is not really suitable for addition to ready-made powders because it tends to make them cake. Moisture is exchanged between the hexametaphosphate and the other ingredients, and if they are at all sensitive to moisture a fine free-flowing powder can be converted into a rock-like mass. Sodium tripolyphosphate is more adaptable for addition to alkaline powders and is almost universally used for the dishwashing detergents on the market.

The softening of water by complex phosphates is achieved by the formation of calcium phosphates which are soluble in water and therefore do not precipitate. The calcium and magnesium are held, or *sequestered,* in a form that does not allow them to react with the alkalis in the dishwashing detergent. It is normally calculated that one part of calcium ion is sequestered by 14 parts by weight of hexametaphosphate, or about 20 parts by weight of hydrated tripolyphosphate. This may also be expressed in the form that one part of calcium carbonate will be sequestered by six parts of hexametaphosphate or eight parts of hydrated tripolyphosphate. If therefore the water has a hardness of 250 p.p.m. as calcium carbonate, it will require about 1/5 ounce per gallon of hexametaphosphate or 1/4 ounce per gallon of tripolyphosphate to soften it. If the powder is designed to be used at 3/4 ounce per gallon of tank capacity, it must contain *at least* 27 per cent hexametaphosphate or 33 per cent tripolyphosphate because the rinsing water which dilutes the detergent will introduce more hardness salts, and there must be a reservoir of softening agent to deal with this. In practice the powder should contain about 50 per cent tripolyphosphate.

The consequence for the dishwashing machine user is obvious. If he is using, say, 50 pounds of dishwashing machine powder per week (a reasonable figure for a large installation) he is actually buying 25 pounds of detergent and 25 pounds of water softener, or about 13 hundredweight per year. The economics of installing an efficient water-softening plant to supply water to the dishwashing machine are very favorable compared with the cost of this amount of water softener, and such a move will give greater improvements in the standards of dishwashing than any juggling with the type or amount of detergent used in hard water. A straightforward zeolite plant can be fitted in a small space, and requires very little in the way of servicing.

One further ingredient of dishwashing powders may be mentioned: sodium aluminate is included in most of the products to protect the glaze and color of good china. It is not sufficiently realized that the glaze of china, though hard and resistant, can be damaged by detergents or even soap in very hot water, such as is used in dishwashing machines, and in the case of the finest china, in which decoration is applied over the glaze, color can be removed. This is not a problem that will concern most industrial caterers, but the precaution of adding sodium aluminate costs very little.

### Rinse Aids

Even with the most efficient detergent, the dishes may be left with traces of food material, starch from potatoes and so on, loosely adhering to the surface. Because the volume of rinsing water is kept low in most machines, to reduce the dilution of the detergent tank, it is possible for the last drops of rinse to contain such food residues when they dry on the plate, and unsightly marks are left. In hard water these effects are more pronounced, and the combined effect of hard water and dirty detergent solution can leave plates and glassware with streaks and spots. Intelligent operation of the machine should obviate these troubles, but every manager knows that intelligent use cannot be guaranteed. A precaution against such troubles is the inclusion in the rinse water of a very small amount of wetting agent, to make sure that the water drains away completely from the work before it has a chance to dry.

Such a wetting agent must be quite safe, in the sense that it is non-toxic and cannot taint the work, and it must be completely non-foaming, because the agitation in the rinse sprays of the machine is very fierce. The wetting agent can be introduced into the rinse line with a simple venturi device, and most machine suppliers will fit a suitable injector. In general the use of a rinse aid is a reasonable precaution against careless use of the machine, but the installation of soft water will do much to make this unnecessary.

## TYPES OF JET MACHINE

### SMALL MACHINES

For the caterer who is concerned with a fairly small quantity of meals, less than 300 per hour maximum, for example, a machine without mechanical conveyers may be quite satisfactory. In all these, the trays are put into the machine by hand, the machine performs a wash and rinse cycle to a preset pattern, then switches off and the tray is removed.

These smaller machines may be divided into three classes with increasing capacities for work:

1. Machines with integral rack systems
2. Hood machines
3. Door machines

### MACHINES WITH INTEGRAL RACK SYSTEMS

These machines are similar to most of the household dishwashing machines in that they have a system of racks fitted permanently into the washing cabinet, and dishes and cutlery are taken to the machine for loading, rather than being loaded into trays at the point of use. This means that the machine cannot be used while loading and unloading are going on, and they are therefore only suitable for a fairly light load of work. One well-known make has a free-standing cabinet machine fitted with a plate rack which can hold 16 large plates or 24 side plates, plus a cup or glass rack with capacity for 15 pieces.

After the machine has been loaded, the door is closed and this automatically switches on the jets to give a washing cycle of 135 seconds with detergent solution, 30 seconds drain, fill with clean water (15 seconds) and 30 seconds rinse. The total cycle is thus 3 1/2 minutes. The manufacturers claim a work output of 375 dishes or 675 glasses per hour, but obviously the rate-controlling factor is the speed of reloading, and these figures presuppose a very active operator for the machine. A practical figure would probably be about 50 meals per hour.

HOOD MACHINES

In these machines, standard racks or trays are used, usually 16" x 16" or 20" x 20", and these can be loaded and unloaded while the machine is in operation on another tray. The operator opens the machine, takes out the rack of washed work, pushes in another rack and switches on for the wash cycle. The characteristic of hood machines is that they have a top in the form of a semicircular hood, and the wash and rinse jets work from under the tray, jets bouncing off the hood to give washing from the top. Figure 10.2 shows the principle.

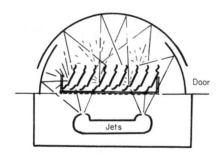

Figure 10.2

Hood type dishwashing machine.

Hood dishwashers can be used for outputs of up to 1000 pieces per hour, or even a little more with well-trained personnel. The wash cycle is usually about 45-60 seconds, then the work is rinsed.

DOOR MACHINES

In these, the work is loaded into trays in the same way as for hood machines, but the washing is done by jets above and below the trays. The entry to the machine is usually provided by lift-up doors which permit the trays to be pushed in. As the doors close again the jets are automatically switched on for the wash cycle, and opening the door switches off the water, so as to save careless personnel from scalding themselves or flooding the kitchen. Most models are supplied "straight through," where the trays enter on one side and leave on the opposite side, but most manufacturers also supply a corner model, where the doors are at right angles and the machine can fit into a corner of the kitchen. These machines can usually deal with up to 3000 pieces per hour.

CONVEYER MACHINES

When the number of pieces exceeds 3000 per hour, or about 300 full meals per hour, a conveyer machine becomes necessary. The delays due to waiting time in the smaller machines become too great to be tolerated, and it becomes necessary to invest in a machine that keeps the trays moving all the time.

As will have been clear from the section describing the principles of the jet dishwasher, the main problem is to attain the desired degree of cleanliness in the shortest possible time, and to keep the detergent solution in a fit state for cleaning as long as possible. In a large machine, in a busy kitchen, the speed may be very high indeed, and the amount of debris left on the plates would soon soil the detergent solution to such an extent that it would be useless as a cleanser. Rinse-water, in some machines, dilutes the detergent and may float off some of the soiling, but for the best effect it is necessary to divide the washing process into several different stages and keep the water supply and drainage separate. The medium-sized machines incorporate two of these, and the larger machines incorporate others. The ideal washing process may be outlined as follows:

1. *Scrapping section:* This removes gross soiling from plates, and residues of coffee and other drinks from cups. For economy this section can be supplied with soiled water left over from the rinsing section further along the machine. Temperature is not critical as long as it is not too high, but pressure should be high. Drainage is straight to outlet, through a suitable strainer, assuming a satisfactory grease-trap in the drainage system.
2. *Main wash section* This is the pressure/detergent combination that carries out most of the washing. With a prewash scrapping section, the detergent tank should stay wholesome for quite a long time.
3. *Power rinse section:* This washes off the detergent solution and any remaining starchy material, etc. The temperature of the rinse should be about 160° F (70° C) so that the dishes are heated up before the final rinse, but the water is not hot enough to cause hardening of any residual protein in the surface water left from the detergent tank. Water from the power rinse section can be used to make up the prewash, or to dilute the detergent tank by steady degrees.

4. *Hot rinse section:* This should be a fine spray of water at least 180° F (82° C) which sterilizes the work and makes it hot enough to dry in air.

5. *Air drying section:* This is only required for melamine and similar plastic ware. The plastic has a lower specific heat than china, and does not therefore retain quite enough heat from the rinse section to dry spontaneously. Most manufacturers of dishwashing machines will fit an air drying section for plactic ware.

Medium-sized machines usually have only the detergent wash section and the hot rinse section; these will give an output of about 6000 pieces per hour. With scrapping and power rinse added, output can go up to 10,000 pieces per hour.

ROTARY MACHINES

With a large machine handling 10,000 pieces per hour, it is obvious that the mechanical details of loading so many articles and getting the trays to the machine will become a major matter of concern. One solution to this problem is to fit the machine with a specially designed table which runs from the outlet back to the inlet (see Figure 10.3). Trays of dishes

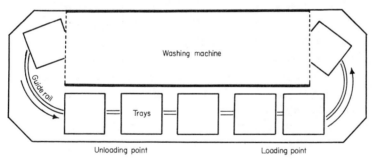

Figure 10.3

Rotary dishwashing machine: layout.

which have left the machine are guided to the working table, where they are emptied and the clean work stacked away. As soon as each tray is emptied, another operator loads up with dirty dishes and the tray is automatically taken back into the machine. The machines are fitted with a conveyer that extends through the whole system.

FLIGHT-TYPE MACHINES

For the large outputs considered above, the other alternative is to eliminate trays altogether, and provide a continuous conveyer onto which the work can be loaded directly. A feature of these machines is the conveyer, which is either a series of perforated V-shaped pockets or a conveyer with pegs to hold the work. This conveyer extends out of the washing area of the machine to give space for loading and unloading, so the machines are quite long, usually 14-25 feet. Of course, a conventional machine would have to have tables for the trays, so there is not so much difference in the space needed.

## GLASS WASHERS

For snack bars, drug stores, and similar establishments having a large trade in cold drinks served in glasses, a specialized glass washer may be a better investment than a conventional dishwasher. The smaller models have cradles in a permanent rack system, so that the glasses are loaded at the front of the machine, which is then closed, and the racks circulate through jets of detergent and a hot rinse section.

For the larger establishment the glasses are loaded into wire trays which can also be used for permanent storage, and these trays travel through the machine in the same way as in a conveyer dishwashing machine.

In washing glasses, the value of soft water will be even more apparent than in dishwashing. However carefully the detergent is formulated, the use of alkalis in hard water is an attempt to do two diametrically opposite things—to clean all debris from a glass with a detergent that is itself creating a solid precipitate in the water. The installation of a water softener is not a major capital item for glass washing machines, as even a large glass washer uses only about 120 gallons of water per hour when running continuously.

It may be useful to point out here that alkali in soft water is the best medium for washing beer glasses in particular. The head of beer, which is stabilized by proteins in the drink (derived from the malt) seems to be very easily affected by traces of other foaming agents, many of which interfere with the protein foam. The traces of detergent that can cause this are very small indeed, and glasses that have been quite carefully rinsed can still cause trouble, as detergent materials can be *adsorbed* onto the surface of the glass.

Sodium dodecyl benzene sulfonate, which is the basis of many liquid detergents, is rather troublesome in this respect. Unfortunately the organic alternatives are all rather high-priced detergents, and the use of a plain alkaline solution in soft water will be found to be by far the best solution.

## VENDING MACHINES

The growing cost of catering personnel, especially for part-time work such as serving coffee in offices and so on, has led to an enormous increase in the number of vending machines serving beverages and meals. There are large numbers of these machines also in public places, serving milk and other commodities.

The usefulness of these machines cannot be denied, and they will undoubtedly become even more common than they are at present, and serve even more complicated foodstuffs. The great disadvantage of them is not one that is inherent in the mechanism, but in the attitude of people towards them.

The supplies that go into a vending machine are very carefully packaged goods; the coffee is a special concentrate, the meals are packed in the most modern plastic materials, the milk is cartoned in a package that will retain the pasteurized condition of the contents, and cooled to a safe temperature. Everything suggests, in fact, that the foodstuffs in a vending machine do not require the same hygienic care as the same foodstuffs in a more "open" condition—they are just so many packets in the machine, just as if they were packs of cigarettes or envelopes of nylons. This attitude can give rise to staggering examples of negligence in hygiene, like the milk vending machine that was returned to the manufacturers as having a faulty mechanism. The manufacturers found that the moving parts, including the coin mechanism, were thickly crusted with old sour milk and mold growing a quarter of an inch thick. It seems incredible that anyone should allow any milk vessel to get into this condition, but the "packeted" milk was obviously regarded as something different, and outside the normal rules of hygiene.

The problem with most vending machines is a multiple one:

1. The machine is usually some way from a supply of water, so it is necessary to bring cleaning solution to it.
2. Cleaning employees might easily be able to clean the machine, but the contents—money and negotiable goods—may give rise to reluctance that they should have a key to the machine.
3. The authorized machine service man may be a visiting agent who has little time to deal with the hygienic aspects of the job.
4. Any detergent used must be quite safe with all the materials of construction, otherwise the coin mechanism or other moving parts may be corroded.
5. If the same person is filling the machine, taking out the money, and cleaning the inside of the machine, there may be a serious hygiene problem, especially as he or she may not easily be able to wash between visits.
6. Any detergent used must be odorless and unable to taint or spoil food and drink in the machine.

The obvious answer is a germicidal detergent, so that risk of contamination by the person servicing the machine will be reduced, but several of the common germicides are ruled out. Phenols and chlorinated phenols have too strong a smell to be used in close contact with food, especially as it is unlikely that the solution will be rinsed off the inside surfaces of the machine. Sodium hypochlorite would be too corrosive for metals, formaldehyde and ethylene oxide are too dangerous for use by unskilled personnel, complex phenols and similar materials are too expensive and not sufficiently active against molds and yeasts.

The best solution is a cationic germicide. Quaternary ammonium compounds such as benzalkonium chloride are quite effective, have very little taste or smell at working concentrations, are not corrosive and are pleasant to use. Even better is the chlorhexidine type of germicide, which has better action against molds and yeasts as well as bacteria, and operators of vending machines are well advised to use either 1 per cent chlorhexidine digluconate or 2 per cent benzalkonium chloride.

Such a solution should be carried around by the vending machine service man in a plastic bottle with a sponge for application. Alternatively, one of the proprietary applicators may be used. The solution should be rubbed freely over all the parts of the machine, taking special care to remove any spilled milk or sugary solutions (a small nylon pad is useful for this purpose) and any excess of solution wiped up with a paper towel, which is discarded after treating each machine. There is no need to rinse, as the solutions are not corrosive and the trace of germicide left on the metal will help to combat contamination. Such a small kit is easy to carry and does not involve very much thought or effort on the part of the operator, so there is every hope that it will be used, where a larger and more elaborate cleaning kit would probably be left in the truck.

In offices where the machine is filled by maintenance personnel, the same sort of kit can be kept handy to the machine or machines, and used solely for them by the person authorized to fill the machine and collect the money.

# eleven

# Washrooms

Because of the intimate connection between personal hygiene and the washroom, the standards in this part of the building are viewed with a far more critical eye than any other. An office worker who does not apparently notice or care that there is dust on his filing cabinet or a coffee stain on his carpet will complain bitterly if the washbasin is dirty or the toilet stained. The maintenance manager must therefore resign himself to the fact that his efficiency will be judged by the condition of the washrooms, and make sure that they reflect the standards of hygiene he is trying to achieve in other parts of the building.

There is, fortunately, an unexpected bonus to be gained from special care of the washrooms. There is no doubt (whatever the psychology may be) that people reflect the standards of the washroom in their own behavior. A dirty or neglected washroom seems an irresistible invitation to vandalism and dirty habits; conversely, a clean, bright, convenient washroom may actually encourage better standards of hygiene and behavior among its users.

## SOAPS

If we desire to raise the standards of hygiene in our offices and plants, it is essential that people should be given every encouragement to wash their hands more often. Every surface is covered with germs of various kinds, and many of these are more or less pathogenic. The skin is occupied by germs that are harmful if taken internally, and the nose by germs that can cause skin eruptions. The bowel is a breeding ground for uncountable numbers of bacteria, and many of these are extremely dangerous if introduced into food. Too few people, even now, realize how little protection is offered by ordinary toilet paper against contamination of the hands by these bacteria.

Ideally, every lavatory should be designed so that it is almost impossible to leave it without being reminded of the washbasin. Most maintenance managers have to accept the layout they have already, but they can do their best to make washing attractive by provision of hot water, soap, and drying facilities—without all three, most users do not bother to wash their hands.

Toilet soap bars of the 2½–3 ounce size are convenient to the hand and offer reasonable economy in use. The standards laid down in Chapter Two should be followed in selecting the soap. Perfume and color are a matter of choice, except that it should be realized that the cost of the perfume in a domestic-type toilet soap cake is quite a significant part of the raw materials cost, and therefore a highly-perfumed bar will cost more than one with less perfume. This is a matter of basic cost, not the manufacturers' profit margin. Women workers, by tradition, like a soap with a reasonable level of perfume, and the extra cost paid for this may be considered a tolerable insurance against complaints. It is almost incredible to anyone who has not studied the soap trade from the inside to find how often a soap with a pleasant perfume is described by users as mild, foamy, and smooth, while the same soap without perfume is harsh, will not lather, and gritty in texture—according to the reports of quite intelligent users. Men, if asked outright, will usually say with some emphasis that they dislike a soap with a strong perfume, but in practice they use the same kinds of soap as women and show the same preferences.

The use of germicidal toilet soaps is very attractive as an extra aid to hygiene, and soaps containing about 0.15–0.2 per cent of Vancide BN or one of the related germicides are in fact fairly effective in reducing skin bacterial numbers. Such soaps would certainly encourage hygiene in industries where food is handled, or where food is handled, or where an extra degree of hygiene is necessary for other reasons. In the food trade, the perfume level of soap should be kept low so as to avoid tainting of food with unwanted odors, but it is not necessary to use an entirely unperfumed soap. The types of perfumery material that are really persistent on the skin are not much used in soap perfumes and not at all in the cheaper types of toilet soap, and a small amount of perfume is desirable for the reasons already stated.

## LIQUID SOAPS

The toilet soap bar, in use in lavatories, has two disadvantages: some people object to using a communal bar (usually because it is sometimes left dirty), and bars are pilfered. The best answer to both these problems is to use a liquid toilet soap with an effective dispenser. Each person receives his or her ration of soap without contact with that used by the previous person, and the product is difficult to pilfer from the dispensers and even more difficult to remove from the building. The simplest type of dispenser installation is liquid potash soap, as described in Chapter Two, in a tip-up dispenser. These devices all depend on the partial vacuum created by pouring out soap from a small nozzle in an otherwise closed container to dispense a small quantity of liquid, after which the dispenser has to be allowed to return to its upright position and tilted again before more soap can be obtained. The dispensers are available in glass and various plastics.

Tip-up dispensers require a fairly liquid consistency in the soap, otherwise they will not deliver at all, and "runny" liquid is not always favorably received by users. It seems to have none of the smooth, lubricant qualities of normal soap. They possess another disadvantage also, because the soap tends to dry up in the small nozzle and there is no positive force to clear it; the nozzles have to be poked out or (preferably) washed in hot water at fairly frequent intervals. The type of soap used in these dispensers is usually, because of the viscosity limitation, a potassium soap of coconut, palm kernel, or cheaper fats, and these soaps tend to be irritating to the skin and may, in the cheaper varieties, leave a very unpleasant odor on the skin even after rinsing. The low viscosity necessary could be achieved in other ways (by, for instance, adding alcohol in small quantities to a potassium tallow soap), but this would make the problem of drying-out more acute. It must be accepted, in fact, that the tip-up dispenser only lends itself to a rather inferior type of product.

Better products can be used, under more positive control, by installing dispensers with a positive piston action to expel the soap. In most of these, pushing up the nozzle works a piston which delivers a predetermined quantity of soap. If liquid soap at about 20 per cent total fatty matter (22 per cent soap) is used, one dispenser containing two pints will give about 360 washes, or (as one dispenser can usually serve about 25 people satisfactorily) about five days' use.

All dispensers of every kind should be very robust against rough usage and vandalism. It is important that no washroom fixtures should have fixing screws or nuts that are easily accessible to the casual screwdriver or wrench, and the product inself should only be accessible to authorized persons.

For larger installations, the wash fountain with multiple dispensing points is a convenient way of serving a large number of personnel in a short time; alternatively, the washroom can be fitted with a centralized reservoir system carrying soap from a tank to points by the wash basins.

The care of a well-designed piston-type dispenser is simple. The reservoir should be kept well filled, so that the product cannot dry or thicken in the lower parts of the reservoir or the valve mechanism, and whenever possible the dispensers should be emptied altogether and washed through with hot water. If a dispenser should happen to become clogged with soap, a small amount of alcohol poured into the bottom of the reservoir will usually clear it away rapidly. No lubrication of the valves is necessary, as the soap performs this function admirably.

POWDERED SOAPS

Another method of avoiding the pilferage of soap bars is to dispense the soap in the form of a powder. The powders on the market are usually made from the same fat content as ordinary toilet soap, but dried to a greater extent to prevent the possibility of caking or stickiness. Perfume added to such powders tends to evaporate or spoil rather quickly because of the large surface exposed to the air, and therefore many of the commercial products are unperfumed.

It must be said that, whatever the merits of the soaps actually used, powdered hand soaps of this kind are not very popular with the users. The drying of the soap, which is necessary to avoid clogging in the dispenser, makes the powders rather slow to dissolve and either gritty or sticky on the wet hands, and many users refuse to believe that the quality of the soap is as good as that in a bar of toilet soap. It seems that they equate it with kitchen soap or washing powders.

Another type of powder dispenser actually grates soap from a suitably shaped bar: the same objections, or prejudices, apply to this method also.

## HAND CLEANSERS

Under many circumstances, ordinary soap and water are inadequate to remove the dirt from grease, lubricating oil, graphite, and so on. Such problems used to be confined to the engineering and heavy industries, but it is a curious fact that the growing mechanization and complexity of office work has actually increased the numbers of jobs that are "dirty," at least sometimes—duplicators, photocopiers, litho machines and so on, are all liable to produce dirt that is too heavy for soap and water.

The most effective treatment for most of this dirt is solvent, and white spirit is probably the most suitable material. It is a good solvent for grease and oil, and many materials such as printing ink; it is fairly harmless to the skin, apart from a certain drying action if it is used too frequently; and it is cheap. However, white spirit alone would be difficult to use safely, and dispensers containing the solvent alone would be a fire hazard. It is possible to make a jelly-like material by emulsifying white spirit in soap solution, and adding small amounts of phenol or cyclohexanol or similar materials to clarify the emulsion. The droplets of white spirit in the emulsion become so small that they no longer scatter light, and therefore the emulsion passes from a creamy appearance to an almost transparent jelly. This also has the advantage that the soap solution helps to wash the mixture of white spirit and grease off the hands after the jelly has been rubbed on.

There are many jelly cleansers of this type on the market, all based on the same sort of formula, and they can be purchased in small containers for individual use (by dipping the fingers in) or in large units. The dipping method is wasteful, especially if the consistency of the product allows users to take out a large handful, and it is better to use the large containers and a suitable dispenser. The piston type, modified for the product, is obviously the only practicable dispenser, as gravity feed would be very slow. Many of the suppliers of the cleansing jellies can also supply a dispenser, using materials that are not subject to corrosion or solvent action.

The white spirit emulsions are penetrating compounds, sharing as they do the solvent powers of petroleum spirit and the setting powers of soap solution, and the jellies act as quite efficient paint strippers, and also swell some plastics. It is important therefore that there should be no painted doors or other obstructions between the jelly dispenser and the wash basins (trouble of this kind arises, for instance, in machine shops where operators have small tins of jelly cleanser by their machines, and start to apply this on their way to the washroom so as to save time. Any painted doors along their path will soon be stripped of paint where the hands touch them).

## NON-SOLVENT CLEANSERS

An alternative to white spirit, for less heavy dirt, is to make use of the grease-removing powers of the nonionic detergents. Concentrated nonionics such as nonylphenol condensates will remove grease from the hands quite efficiently if rubbed on full strength and then rinsed off with warm water, and dilutions of this type of detergent, with the addition of a small amount of soap, alcohol to assist in dissolving the soap, and perfume, are sold as hand cleansers. For many purposes the nonionic detergent by itself is cheaper. They are less drying to the skin than white spirit or similar solvents, but not quite as fast or thorough in removing grease.

Alternatively and most cheaply, mixtures of dry soap powder and powdered borax crystals are used as hand cleansers. Borax is a mild alkali, and has some powers of grease removal (though not for the mineral oils and greases which form the greater part of engineering dirt) and the crystals, before they dissolve in water, form a mild abrasive that helps to scour off the heavier dirt. The mixtures are not very pleasant to use, and have little to recommend them except their low price. The same objections apply to the powdered soaps for hand washing. Similar mixtures, using powdered soap and wood flour or other mild abrasives, used to be sold widely, but user reaction against them has virtually removed them from the market.

### GERMICIDAL CLEANSERS

Too little attention has been paid to the possibility of adding an effective germicide to hand cleansers. The need is obvious. In industries where these heavy-duty cleansers are necessary, cuts and abrasions to the hands are common, and these wounds can easily become infected, leading to lost time and other serious consequences. The method of use of solvent jelly and nonionic hand cleansers is very favorable to the use of a germicide, because the products are rubbed into the skin in the concentrated form, and therefore the germicide is not very much diluted with water until the washing-off stage. Under these conditions, about 0.15-0.2 per cent of Vancide BN will be effective in limiting the numbers of bacteria on the skin, especially *Staphylococci.*

## BARRIER CREAMS

Barrier creams are designed to offer some protection to the skin against irritating or contaminating materials used in the course of work. They fall into two classes, dry work creams and wet work creams.

Dry work barrier creams are intended to prevent undue soiling of the skin by dirt, grease, tar, dyestuffs, or other contaminating materials, by covering the skin with a layer of cream that will be an effective barrier to the contaminant, and that can be washed off, with the contaminant, after work. They are usually made with a basic mixture of soap and a filler, such as kaolin, and various other materials added to improve the consistency of the cream and ward off certain specialized soilings. It is fairly obvious that such a cream must be very adherent to the skin if it is to withstand flexing at the knuckles and similar joints, and in fact these regions usually become starved of the cream shortly after application, and tend to pick up contamination even when the rest of the hand is protected. For this reason, barrier creams should not be expected to perform the same function as rubber gloves—shielding the hand against really dangerous materials. With this limitation, a dry work cream containing about 20 per cent kaolin, 5 per cent soap and 8 per cent other fatty material (lanolin, acetyl alcohol, petroleum jelly, or a mixture of these) will protect the hands reasonably well against dust, tar, and similar materials, and will wash off after work, preferably using a liquid hand cleanser of the nonionic type, leaving the hands smooth and clean.

Such a mixture may tend to separate during storage, and appear as a layer of soapy liquid floating on a mass of filler. Stirring will reconstitute the mixture quite well, but the effect is unesthetic. Manufacturers tend to add gums or emulsifiers (methyl cellulose, nonionic emulsifiers and other materials) to stabilize the products.

Wet work barrier creams for use with water and aqueous solutions present a far greater problem in formulation. The product has to satisfy two almost diametrically opposed requirements. It must protect the skin, all day if necessary, against the penetration of water and any harmful materials the water may carry with it, including alkalis and other cleansing agents, yet it must come off the hands after work with ordinary cleansing agents in water. For really stringent conditions, of course, the hands could be covered with a material like nitrocellulose, which requires a solvent to remove it, but rubber or polythene gloves would serve the purpose better and avoid the drying effect of the solvent on the skin.

The best compromise is a mixture of fatty material such as petroleum jelly, lanolin (added mainly to make the product more adherent to the skin), a small amount of emulsifier (but as little as is necessary for the stability of the product, because emulsifier will inevitably allow the cream to become wetted more easily) and a metalic soap such as zinc stearate or magnesium stearate. These materials are, chemically, soaps, but as they are insoluble in water they tend to behave far more as very adherent fatty substances. The addition of silicones to such a mixture adds tremendously to the water resistance, and for very stringent conditions silicone oil should be present at levels of 5 per cent or more. Quite effective wet work barriers can be made with silicone fluids, emulsifier, and water alone, but the cost is rather high.

Such creams are of necessity difficult to remove by ordinary washing methods, and a solvent jelly type of cleanser will be necessary.

Barrier creams for specific use against solvents may be made with such gums as triethanolamine alginate, polyvinylpyrrolidone or methyl cellulose. Such materials are quite harmless to the skin, easy to remove with soap and water, but impervious to trichloroethylene and similar solvents. They offer valuable protection against drying and defatting of the skin in such operations as solvent degreasing of small parts, and similar work.

Barrier creams for use in high temperature conditions, such as furnace rooms, smelters, or radiation from arc lamps and similar light sources, are usually made of a silicone-based wet work cream with the addition of a masking agent such as titanium dioxide at about 30 per cent, tinted to avoid the startling whiteness of the basic formula.

All barrier creams tend to be thick and viscous, as they are designed to adhere to surfaces. Most of the conventional dispensers are therefore too slow in operation when filled with barrier cream, and many may be clogged up altogether. The ideal dispenser is one that forces the cream out by pressure applied from above (like toothpaste from a tube), and very satisfactory screw-operated dispensers are on the market. For many creams, a "follower plate" resting on the surface of the cream will help to maintain an even flow of product. (See Figure 11.1.)

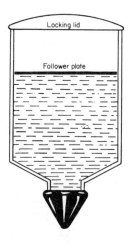

Figure 11.1

Use of follower plate in dispensers for creams, etc.

## TOILETS AND URINALS

"Washroom" is a euphemism for the most important purpose of this part of a building, and the maintenance and hygiene of toilets and urinals is most important for esthetic as well as health reasons. In both cases, the problems are twofold. The equipment is subject to constant running water or water standing open to the air, and the excretions which pass through the equipment are a primary source of staining, odors and health hazards.

The ordinary toilet bowl can be soiled in several ways. Hardness in the water supply can cause deposits of lime or magnesia in the form of a scale on the porcelain, which can easily build up in the idle period when the water in the pan is left slowly evaporating. Iron in the water supply can cause brownish stains, which are exaggerated if there is already lime scale to pick up the dissolved iron salts, and copper from copper or brass plumbing can cause green stains which are also picked up by the lime. Fecal matter may be left on the side of the bowl or accumulate in the bottom of it if the flushing water is not very powerful, and again the roughness caused by deposited lime will make the conditions worse. Lastly, rubbish of various kinds is often discarded into the bowl, and some of this may give rise to staining.

The common toilet brush is a useful means of clearing some types of soiling, but is in itself a most unhygienic object, as it is almost impossible to decontaminate the bristles effectively. Proper hygiene, therefore, requires that the bowl should be cleansed thoroughly with as little mechanical help as possible.

## ACID CLEANSERS

Lime, magnesia, iron and copper stains can all be dissolved away with acids, and hydrochloric acid (muriatic acid) has been used for this purpose for many years. However, it is rather a dangerous material to handle, as splashing may cause irritation to the skin and could cause serious damage to the eyes. The dangers of breakage, if the acid is kept in bottles, are also considerable, and costly corrosion could follow the spilling of a quantity of the acid in a storeroom or similar premises.

Almost as effective, and far less dangerous, is sodium bisulfate, a solid crystalline compound which could be described as halfway between neutral sodium sulfate and sulfuric acid. It has most of the acidity of sulfuric acid without the inconvenience of being liquid. A crude form of sodium bisulfate called niter cake (once a by-product of the production of nitric acid from Chile niter) is quite satisfactory for toilet cleansing. This is used, with perfume, in most of the heavy crystalline powders sold as toilet cleansers. In ordinary use it should be shaken into the bowl and left, preferably for about 12 hours, and then flushed away. It can also be used as a kind of scouring powder to remove iron and copper stains from the sides of the bowl and from the vertical surfaces of urinals.

Sodium bisulfate (or other acids) has little effect on fecal stains and very little germicidal action. As a hygiene measure it is therefore very limited.

CHLORINATED CLEANSERS

Sodium hypochlorite and the other sources of chlorine described in Chapter Two can all be used to bleach fecal stains, and chlorine is, of course, an excellent germicide for the water in the bowl. Unfortunately chlorine has no effect on lime or iron stains. Indeed, sodium hypochlorite, which is usually rather alkaline for stabilization, can precipitate more lime or magnesia from hard water. The aim should be to create conditions of about 60 p.p.m. of available chlorine in the water remaining in the bowl. As the average content is about 1/2 gallon of water, about 1.2 c.c. of 10 per cent hypochlorite is sufficient for bacterial killing, and most users would add far more than this.

If sodium hypochlorite is mixed with acid, it yields free chlorine gas. Under controlled conditions this may be an excellent way of removing stains, but if the quantities of both materials are quite large, a dangerous concentration of the gas may be swept out of the bowl into the face of the operator; this is distressing and may be harmful to lungs and eyes. For this reason it is unwise to mix different types of toilet cleanser.

A better method of maintaining hygiene and cleanliness in washrooms is to issue sodium hypochlorite solution for daily cleaning of toilet bowls, and make a special addition of a sodium bisulfate cleanser before the weekend, after the chlorinating agent has had a chance to wear off. The acid cleanser will keep the bowls free of lime, and the daily treatment with hypochlorite will maintain a high standard of bacteriological hygiene. Urinals can be treated the same way, except that if there is a suspicion of iron or copper staining from the pipework, the powder can be brushed over the vertical surface of the urinal and allowed to fall into the channel and over the edge tiles.

CHANNEL BLOCKS

A popular aid to hygiene in washrooms are the so-called "channel blocks." These are small blocks of perfumed material which are scattered in the channels of urinals or fixed in the toilet bowl so as to be washed over by the flushing water. Similar blocks are sold, for fitting into suitable holders, as deodorants for the toilet.

All these blocks are made of para-dichlorobenzene, a crystalline organic material derived from coal tar or petroleum benzene. It has a powerful, not unpleasant smell, and the interesting property that it *sublimes* (i.e. when it is heated or exposed to air, it does not melt to a liquid, but evaporates straight to a vapor. Camphor and iodine are other materials with this property). This sublimation makes it useful for such purposes as moth rings, because, in the warm environment of the clothes closet, the crystals evaporate into every part of the closet without producing any liquid which could run over the linen or clothes stored there. Similarly, a block of para-dichlorobenzene stored in a washroom will evaporate slowly, spreading its odor around without melting and possibly blocking up the drain or spilling on the floor. The blocks are usually wrapped in cellophane for storage, and this material has a tendency to crack in tiny pinholes at the corners and other folds. The pinholes allow the para-dichlorobenzene to sublimate, and therefore it is quite common to find small pits or holes in the blocks just under the corners. Para-dichlorobenzene is not soluble in water to any extent that is significant, so the blocks can be kept in conditions of running water without undue losses.

For the purposes of deodorant blocks and the better kind of channel block, perfumes are usually added to increase the covering power for other odors. The cheapest method of use, at the other extreme, is to buy plain crystals of para-dichlorobenzene and scatter these about.

While the smell of the product is (to most people) pleasant and associated with hygiene, and the perfumed blocks can cover up the unpleasant washroom smells very well, two things must be understood about these blocks. Para-dichlorobenzene has no true *deodorant* effect—it has no chemical or other effect on the sources of the odors, but only masks them with a stronger smell of its own; it has absolutely no effect on bacteria or other micro-organisms. It is therefore in no way a substitute for adequate cleaning and sanitizing of the washroom and its fittings.

Para-dichlorobenzene, like other similar chlorinated aromatic compounds, is quite a good solvent, and the crystals or blocks should not be placed in contact with, or even very near, paintwork, varnished wood, or similar surfaces, because they will eventually soften the paint or varnish. They should not be stored anywhere near foodstuffs, painted or printed material, or varnished goods, as the vapor can escape even from closed packages. They should not be stored anywhere near radiators or other sources of heat, otherwise losses may be extensive. The blocks are usually made in circles or large cubical blocks for urinal drains and in oblong or circular blocks with holes in them for clipping with wire clips to the sides of toilet bowls.

## SANITIZING LIQUIDS

It is common to fit devices to the toilet system which inject a small amount of sanitizing liquid into the flushing water every time the cistern is flushed. This ensures that a fresh charge of germicide is added to the water in the bowl after every use. Such a system would obviously be highly desirable from the point of view of hygiene, if the germicide is added at a level sufficient to kill all or most of the bacteria in the bowl. Unfortunately there are two opposing requirements to such a system:

1. It should be effective against the resident bacteria;
2. It should be economical of sanitizing liquid so that the cost of materials and refilling is reduced to the minimum.

The dosage is usually heavily weighted towards the second requirement, and against the first. Using a highly effective sanitizer like sodium hypochlorite (10 per cent available chlorine), about $1.5$ cm$^3$ per flushing would be required to kill the bacteria in the bowl, so that one pint of the liquid would provide enough sanitizer for about 300 flushes. Using a quaternary ammonium compound, effective against *Escherichia coli* at 5000 p.p.m. (not an unusual figure), one pint would provide only 40 flushes, and many of the phenolic and pine sanitizers provided for these systems are even less effective, so that proper sanitizing would use up a pint of liquid in a few hours. The observed dosage in most of the practical systems would do little more than add a smell of sanitizer to the water.

The same considerations apply to products recommended for use in the water tank itself. Some of these are colored, to show when the product has been exhausted and also to give the impression that *something* is being added to the water. Many dyestuffs give a strong color at only one p.p.m. in water, so it is easier to give the impression of effectiveness than to achieve it in fact.

It has been shown that, in fact, toilet bowls are not a major source of infection as long as they are kept reasonably clean. The number of food poisoning or similar outbreaks traced to this source is negligible, compared with the large number traced to people who did not wash their hands after using the toilet. While the continuous sanitizer systems, therefore, may be an added refinement to a washroom, they should not be allowed to instill a false sense of security in the maintenance staff.

SANITARY NAPKIN DISPOSAL

In any washroom used by female employees, it is advisable to install a suitable disposal unit for sanitary napkins and similar debris from personal hygiene. The alternative, sooner or later, is sure to be an embarrassing blockage in the sewage disposal system.

There are many designs of incinerator on the market, powered by electricity or gas, and capable of reducing sanitary napkins to ashes in a few seconds or minutes. They all require a flue to an outside wall, and some models require additional plumbing for a swilling device. In other models the ashes are removed at intervals by the maintenance personnel.

# twelve

# Vehicles

The cleaning of road vehicles often enters into the responsibilities of the maintenance manager, and may extend from the simple task of seeing that one or two company automobiles are kept clean, to the care of a fleet of trucks or vans in a variety of depots or loading points.

Road vehicles become very dirty in use, especially in bad weather, but even under dry conditions they are covered with "traffic film" which consists of the usual dust constituents, with a heavy emphasis on the mineral materials, stuck together with a blend of road tar, diesel fuel, lubricating oil and rubber from tires. This is a very adherent mixture, similar in consistency and imperviousness to the worst type of machine-shop soiling. The tar, oil and rubber components tend to make it water-repellent, and most detergent solutions, if not assisted by mechanical action, just bounce off and leave the film unattacked. For this reason, auto washing methods that depend solely on high-pressure jets to clean off the film are doomed to failure. A suitable brush is invariably needed in addition.

The qualities of the ideal auto-washing detergent may be stated as follows:

1. It must remove and suspend the traffic film, mud, and such things as bird droppings and the resins shed by some trees.
2. It must not damage cellulose paint, plastics, rubber, steel, aluminum or chromium plate.
3. It should easily be rinsed, and leave no solid residue if the rinsing is inadequate. The "streaking" effect should be as little as possible.
4. It should have a property rather hard to define, a "protective colloid" effect on grit and similar hard soiling, so that the particles of grit are surrounded by

a layer of softer material as they are lifted away from the surface, and retain this protective coating as they are rinsed away. This ensures that the brushing which is necessary to remove traffic film does not rub pieces of grit into the cellulose finish, causing scratches. Profuse and thick foam will have this effect to some extent, as the layer of bubbles helps to cushion the automobile finish against the grit, but the addition of materials such as sodium carboxymethyl cellulose or the alkanolamide type of nonionic will have a more positive action. This is a field in which much development is still needed.

5. The detergent should either leave the surface quite clean and smooth, ready for waxing, or deposit a layer of wax during its use. The second effect is obviously time saving, but may be uneconomical in materials.

The shampoos on the market can fairly be said to meet some of these requirements each, the formulas varying according to the quality which seems most important to the manufacturer concerned. Shampoos with very high foaming characteristcs may be formulated with fatty alcohol sulfates such as those used for hair shampoos and carpet cleaning; these satisfy requirements 2, 3, and 5, have some protective action (requirement 4), but are not very effective detergents and therefore fall down on requirement 1—the essential cleaning job.

Blends of anionic detergents with nonionics, such as are used for general-purpose cleaning, are better detergents and satisfy requirement 1, but they tend to allow close contact between the automobile surface and grit, and therefore fail on requirement 4. Addition of a suitable alkanolamide type detergent will improve matters in this respect.

When detergents are used with a high degree of agitation, as in a washing machine, the use of the fatty alcohol sulfate type may cause excessive foaming, and this may make rinsing difficult. It also causes trouble in disposing of the effluent if large numbers of vehicles are washed. In this case the best solution is to use a nonionic detergent as the shampoo base. These detergents have excellent powers of removing traffic film, but do not foam excessively. It will be found that they do not satisfy requirement 4 very well by themselves, but the addition of small amounts of methyl cellulose to the product will give the solution more "body" and give better protective action against grit scratches.

In auto washing by hand, undoubtedly the best tool is the brush that can be fixed to the end of a hose. The dirt and shampoo are kept on the move by the pressure of the water, thus eliminating the possibility of streaks, and the layer of water that is constantly renewed between the brush and the surface of the auto cuts down the contact between grit and the cellulose. Always use cold water, or at the most lukewarm, as hot water tends to dry too quickly, leaving streaks of dirty detergent on the bodywork, and heat also tends to destroy the protective action by thinning out the solution.

Commence on the lower part of the auto, not the roof. This method avoids the great danger of spilling runs of concentrated detergent down the side of the auto, which invariably leads to permanent streaks. The mechanism of these streaks seems to be as follows: traffic grime is in layers, and the lowest layer is firmly embedded so as to be almost a part of the auto finish. There are also layers where traffic film has become mixed with polish used on the auto. It is impossible to remove all these layers, but the ideal system will remove an even amount all over the surface. A streak of concentrated detergent is likely to remove layers lower down than those removed by diluted detergent, so making a permanent streak mark which shows up when the auto is dry. If the auto is washed from the bottom up, any spills of detergent will run into areas which are already wet, and they will therefore be diluted.

There are devices on the market for adding detergent automatically into the hose line. These are mainly venturi devices, similar in principle to the tap proportioners mentioned in Chapter Five. Such a device is a good investment if there are several vehicles to wash. It is important that the brush should go over every part of the vehicle surface, otherwise traffic film will not be removed evenly; the best method is to go over the auto with detergent twice, once mainly horizontally and the second time vertically, and then wash with clean water.

Rinsing can be facilitated by the addition of a very small amount of non-foaming wetting agent to the rinsing water. This helps to insure that the water drains away rapidly, and there is no risk of water spotting on the finish. The addition of Pluronic L 60 or a similar member of the range, at about 0.01 per cent to the final rinse, will ensure rapid, streak-free drying. Assuming that the final rinse is about 10 gallons of water, the usage of Pluronic will be about 4 $cm^3$.

Some products contain wax, which is deposited on the surface of the bodywork during the washing process—these products are known as "wash and wax" shampoos. They usually contain synthetic polish ingredients similar to those used in dry-bright polishes. It is a rather wasteful method of application of wax, as so much of the dressing is washed away with the shampoo.

## MECHANICAL AUTOMOBILE WASHING

When the number of vehicles to be washed per day exceeds three or four, it is well worth considering the installation of a mechanical washing machine. The growth of auto washing as a subsidiary service industry to the gas station trade has led to intense competition between the manufacturers of equipment, and the prices have reached a point where an efficient unit can be bought for less than one human cleaner's annual salary.

Nearly all these units use the same general process. The auto is wetted with detergent solution, using normal auto-shampoo types of formulation, and then passes between revolving brushes which supply the mechanical action. The irregular shapes of automobiles, and the differences in width and height, are compensated by using brushes with very long bristles which are thrown outwards by centrifugal force as the brushes revolve. The filaments may be made of nylon or other fibers, carefully selected to give a soft flailing action without the risk of scratching paintwork. The auto then passes on to a high-pressure spray of clean water which washes off the detergent and dirt. The units vary in the arrangements they make for washing the fronts and backs of autos in addition to the sides and roof. Some have no such provision, and these areas have to be cleaned by hand, while others have "roller" brushes set at right angles to the main brushes, so that the roller starts at the hood of the automobile, rolls over the hood, screen, and roof, and then passes down the rear of the body. This design is obviously more elaborate and expensive, but saves a good deal of hand labor.

The movement of the auto through the unit is achieved by three main methods:

1. The vehicle is driven through slowly.
2. The vehicle is hooked onto a conveyer that draws it slowly through the detergent spray, brushes, and rinsing spray.
3. The vehicle stands still, and the cleaning unit passes over it. Usually a rectangular frame carries brushes and jets; it passes over the auto from front to back, spraying detergent and brushing, and then returns spraying water and brushing.

The first method, self-drive, is obviously the most popular for the service industry, because the owner or driver is acting as cheap labor to take the auto through the system. For those who have to pay for their labor, the mechanical devices are better. The conveyer system is faster, as the vehicles can go through one after another, but the third method, the traveling washer, probably uses the least labor and is the simplest to operate with untrained personnel. The other advantage of the traveling washer is that it can be installed in any bay which is large enough to hold the vehicle plus a foot or two for free space. Vehicles can be backed in and driven out even if the bay is enclosed on three sides, while the conveyer washer needs clear access from both ends.

## COMMERCIAL VEHICLE WASHING

Commercial vehicles—trucks, and so on—vary far more in size and shape than automobiles, and the design of washing equipment therefore has to be more complicated. In general, however, the system of using wide brushes, with the filaments spun out by centrifugal force, is the method of choice, just as with automobiles. Units for cleaning commercial vehicles are usually of the drive-through type or the traveling washer type. The use of conveyers for very large trucks implies a powerful traction system, and it is better to put the vehicles into position for washing by means of their own power. The body washing unit is often coupled with a unit for washing the underside of the vehicle, through high pressure sprays. This type is useful for removing mud and snow, and also removes salt used for snow clearing; this last, if left on, causes serious corrosion, so the washing equipment can pay for itself in saved maintenance.

Tankers, which are often greasy to a greater extent than any other type of commercial vehicle, may need a special layout of the washing equipment to spray them with solvent-based degreasing materials before they enter the normal type of washer. Because of the convex shape of the tank itself, there are often regions which are deeply indented and difficult to reach with brushes unless the filaments are very long.

Railroad cars and similar rolling stock require different treatment from road vehicles, because the main type of soiling on them is iron oxide. Railroad stock with steel-shod wheels use cast-iron brake blocks (it is necessary that the brake blocks should be good conductors of heat, otherwise the frictional heat on braking might expand the steel "tires" of the wheels and loosen them), and iron oxide showers off the brake blocks when they are applied.

There are various special cleansers for this purpose, mostly based on oxalic acid or sulfamic acid, which are good solvents for iron, but the problem of removing this brown soiling is a difficult one. Those with premises near railroads, especially marshalling yards and sidings where a great deal of braking is done, may find that their walls and windows are covered with this brown dust. The best method for removing adherent patches is sodium citrate solution.

# thirteen

# Pests

We tend to think that urban life is only concerned with human beings, and forget the large numbers of other creatures that share the town environment with us—some easily visible, like birds; some more retiring, like rats and mice; some too small to be seen easily, like ants, roaches, and flies; and some always hidden, like death watch beetles and woodworms. All these can cause trouble to the maintenance manager through losses and damage to stores and food, damage to the structure of the building, disfigurement of the building, or danger to hygiene, and steps must be taken to make sure that none of these threats comes into effect.

In many cases the maintenance manager will need expert advice in dealing with these pests, and this chapter makes no attempt to cover all aspects of the subject in detail (which would be the subject of an equally large book on its own). The following notes are intended to describe the main hazards of the various types of pest, and the various treatments that may be of value in combating them.

## BIRDS

Most people count birds among the ornaments of our towns, and many town dwellers see no other kind of wild creature so frequently or in such numbers. However, picturesque though they may be, birds are messy. They excrete haphazardly, they drop nest-building material and feathers, and they can rapidly ruin the appearance of buildings.

They are also a potential hazard to health. Bird droppings dry in the sun and wind, and the dried material breaks down into dust which blows about, into windows and ventilators. One measurement of the contamination caused in this way has shown that, near the fourth floor of a *new* building, not contaminated with bird droppings itself, the powdered excreta from surrounding older buildings produced between 0.03 milligram and 0.18 milligram of uric acid per cubic meter of air. Uric acid was measured because it could only have originated from bird droppings, but the implication is clear that other and even less desirable materials such as bacteria would also have been blowing about in comparable amounts; in any case, the effects of breathing these quantities of uric acid are not known.

Birds are also a physical hazard to aircraft. In the United States, it is estimated, there are about 800 collisions per year between birds and aircraft, and the U.S. Air Force attributes a loss of $10 million every year to such damage.

Farmers, whose losses from bird depredations are the most heavy and directly measurable, tend to favor killing as a method of control, and various materials are available for this purpose. Strychnine, thallium sulfate, sodium fluoride, and sodium fluoracetate have been recommended for mixing with suitable baits. All these substances are also poisonous to man and other animals, and must be handled and spread with the greatest care. Apart from the dangers, there is also the question of public opinion. The public, who do not directly have to pay for the damage that birds do, have a sentimental attachment to them, and the sight of hundreds of dead birds around a factory or office block would probably cause some outcry. Most maintenance managers would be content if the birds will stay away from their own particular buildings, and particularly not nest on them or excrete on them. There are several ways of achieving this end without poisoning.

One simple and effective way is to spread a harmless soft substance on the ledges and other surfaces favored by the birds. This has the effect of frightening them, apparently because they naturally avoid any surface that appears to be yielding or likely to trap their feet. The materials used are in no sense "bird-lines" (sticky substances designed expressly for trapping the birds) but merely a kind of non-drying putty. The materials are usually applied with a caulking gun or from a tube, in bands about 1/2 inch wide and 1/2 inch thick, a short distance from the edge of the sill or ledge. Second or third bands may be necessary for very wide sills, the object being to have a line of repellent every two inches or so, so that the birds cannot have a firm footing on the surface. The sills or ledges should be clean and dry before application, and with this proviso the material will stay soft yet adherent through rain or sun.

When the birds alight at the ledges, they avoid the strips of repellent, and usually stand at the extreme edge. After one visit, birds rarely return to the treated area.

There are also chemical repellents for birds, used mainly for the treatment of seeds, but also useful for discouraging them from coming into certain parts of buildings. Anthraquinone and tetramethyl thiuram disulfide (TMTD) are suitable repellents that do not actually harm the birds. An alternative treatment that has been found useful is to use a mild poison that does not actually kill the birds, but causes temporary distress. Such a typical material consists mainly of 4-aminopyridine hydrochloride. The powder is spread on bread or grain, etc., and the bait scattered around the birds' favorite resorts. After ingesting some of the substance, a proportion of the birds will begin to flap or cry in a way that suggests danger to the others, and all the birds avoid the area. Baiting twice a week around a large airport reduced the gull population from about 30,000 to about 200, without actually killing any of the birds.

4-Aminopyridine is harmless to other animals—and indeed is not lethal to birds—and an adult pig would have to eat about half a pound of the normal baited grain to be in any danger.

Some selectivity is possible with the use of this and other poisons or repellents in different types of bait. Pigeons, for example, will eat from open pans but not from covered feeders, whereas starlings, which are usually regarded as the greatest nuisance of all, will feed from practically any type of container. Many songbirds are not attracted by grain baits but will eat bread, so the use of grain offers some protection for the more attractive and tolerable birds while not hindering action against gulls and starlings.

There are mechanical devices which can prevent the nesting and fouling of birds in crevices and deep embrasures in stone and other buildings. Nylon nets can be fastened across the gaps, or bird-baffles, with lines of blunt projections placed so as to make birds uncomfortable, can be fitted in the gaps.


## RATS

The black rat and the larger and fiercer brown rat are the chief of these pests. Rats live in colonies and are very gregarious, so they tend to move from one district or building to another in droves if they are persecuted by poison or cats, or if they detect the presence of food waste and other attractive things in a new area. As they are very prolific and breed all year round, a building can soon be seriously overrun unless action is taken as soon as rats are detected.

Rats do several million dollars worth of damage *per week* in food supplies alone. They not only steal food, but damage and pollute more than they eat. They cut holes in floors, walls, and roofs, often letting in water and starting building decay in this way, and will burrow among stocks of all kinds—stationery, packed stock, bins, sacks, and bags—leaving a trail of damage and filth behind them.

They carry diseases such as bubonic plague, Weil's disease, trichinosis, dysentery, and dwarf tape worm, and also food poisoning organisms of the *Salmonella* type. Rat bites are extremely infectious, owing to the pathogenic bacteria which they carry on their teeth. Altogether, rats are the least welcome visitors to any premises.

Trapping of rats is sometimes useful for small invasions and for premises of limited size. There are break-back, spring, and cage traps of a wide variety of sizes and shapes.

In some premises poison gas can be used, and this treatment has the advantage of getting into the tunnels, even underground, and carrying the war into the rats' own territory. However, the use of gas is obviously a highly skilled job, and it may not be feasible if the building has many outlets which would have to be made gas-tight. For smaller scale use, there are proprietary powders on the market which give off poison gas when they are placed down holes, the moisture of the earth causing the reaction. All entrances and bolt holes must be stopped up.

Probably the most suitable method for most premises is the laying of poison bait. There are many poisons suitable for killing rats, the most popular being red squill, zinc phosphide, thallium sulfate, and Warfarin, the last being a particularly deadly poison for rats. It is important to note that all these materials are also poisonous to domestic animals and human beings.

While Warfarin was undoubtedly the best rat poison until a few years ago, in all parts of the world there are developing strains of rats which are resistant to the material. These "super-rats," as the newspapers have christened them, are gradually becoming dominant in the rat world. So far no other poison as effective or safe to use as Warfarin has been developed to take its place.

Whichever poison is used, the baiting must be done with care. Rats are reasonably intelligent animals, and are suspicious of changes in their surroundings. If poisoned bait is put down without preparation it may easily be found that only one or two rats have taken it, and the rest, seeing the bodies, have left it alone. Bait without poison must therefore be set out on two or three occasions to allay the rats' suspicions. A very attractive bait can be made with 3 pounds of wheatmeal flour, 4 ounces of sugar and 2 ounces of grated almonds or confectioners' ground almonds. This mixture must be thoroughly blended, preferably without the operators' hands coming into contact with it, as the rats detect the smell of human beings very acutely.

The mixture is laid for two evenings to encourage the rats to feed, and this will also show where most of the rats are feeding. On the third day, the same bait with poison is laid. This particular bait has been found to attract rats even when there is other food available.

In any campaign against rats, the services of an experienced rat exterminator will be found well worthwhile; rats, as has been said, are intelligent and cunning animals, and detect the machinations of their enemies only too easily. A professional operator gets to know the signs of rat runs and favorite feeding places, and can lay his bait with the maximum effect.

The other general precaution against rats is prevention. Garbage bins should be kept securely closed, food waste cleared up immediately, foodstuffs kept in airtight containers or metal bins rather than sacks. The same precautions apply to raw materials that might attract rats—adhesives based on starch, and the like.

## MICE

Mice are not quite such a hazard to health as rats, but are almost equally destructive and dirty, and like rats tend to spoil more than they eat. They respond to the usual rat poisons, and Warfarin or alpha-chloralose are suitable, but it is sometimes difficult to tell where to lay the bait, as mice can live in any nook or cranny, and do not leave droppings to the extent that rats do.

If the holes can be detected, bait similar to that described for rats, poisoned with Warfarin, can be pushed into the holes, which are then plugged with a piece of wood or even a screw of hard paper.

If the holes cannot be detected, the best plan is to bait areas which are suspected, using bait without poison. One or two nights should be sufficient to show where the mice are feeding, and then poisoned bait can be placed in these areas.

## ROACHES

Roaches are members of the *Blattidae* family, all with flattened, beetle-like bodies, long antennae, and a shiny leathery covering. There are three types, the common U.S. roach, and the smaller oriental and German roaches, all of which seem to have spread to most parts of the world.

All the varieties are omnivorous, preferring sweet and starchy foods, but quite ready to eat any kind of food—papers, books, clothing, shoes, bones, and the bodies of other dead insects. They are unpleasant to look at, and and emit a peculiar disgusting smell which they leave behind them on foodstuffs. Like rats and mice, they tend to spoil and foul far more food than they eat, and an invasion of roaches in a larder or food storage room can render the whole contents inedible.

They are nocturnal creatures, and can often only be detected by the mess they make. If roach traces have been found, the only way to confirm their presence is to wait in the dark for an hour or so, and then turn on the lights suddenly: if there are many of the insects, they may even be audible as they scurry about. Treatment consists of baiting the area with molasses; this can be spread on pieces of polythene or greaseproof paper. The best poison to mix with this bait is dieldrin or lindane, although pyrethrum can also be used to flush out the roaches.

Alternative poisons for roaches are sodium fluoride and thallium sulfate. These are far less suitable for use in kitchens than dieldrin, as they are both extremely poisonous to human beings and animals. Thallium sulfate as a roach killer was the subject of an important labeling test case in Texas in 1968: a child died from eating some of the roach killer, and the manufacturers were found liable because they had not declared on the label that there is no known antidote to thallium poisoning. In general, it seems better to use dieldrin or pyrethrum.

## ANTS

Ants are not particularly dangerous or even dirty, but they can be a nuisance if they take to running through a building, and they can contaminate foodstuffs.

When the runs can be seen, apply sodium fluoride (0.5 per cent of the fluoride in a syrup made from 50 parts water and 50 parts refiners' syrup). Dieldrin can also be used as the poison. Some ants seem to prefer a savory diet, and a mixture of cheese sauce and poison has attracted them more than syrup. In either case, keep the baits well out of the way of other food, and do not use outdoors if rain is present or expected. Usually ants carry away a large proportion of the bait to the nest, and therefore the whole colony is poisoned.

Powdered borax is a harmless ant repellent, scattered over the runs and in cracks and so on where the ants enter the building. It does not seem to do more than repel them, and is not as effective as sodium fluoride or dieldrin in getting rid of the nuisance.

## CARPET BEETLES

These insects are found in two main types—the black carpet beetle, about 3/16 inches long, and the varied carpet beetle, about 1/8 inch long—both infesting all woolen material. The grubs are very hairy little creatures which hide in woodwork, behind skirting boards and under furniture. Treatment is as for moth infestation: carpets must be taken up and sprayed on both sides with a good insecticide such as lindane. The source of the grubs is often an old bird's nest in the roof space.

## CLOTHES MOTHS

These insects lay about 200 eggs at a time, which hatch out into grubs in about 7-10 days; the grubs attack wool for preference, but have also been found to eat mixtures of wool with rayon and other synthetic fibers. The eggs are normally laid in parts of upholstery or garments that are shaded from the light, and there is a preference for soiled portions of the fabric. This is because the grubs need Vitamin B as well as the protein from the wool; the vitamin occurs in such soiling as perspiration. They are most active if the temperature is fairly warm, 70-80° F (20-26° C) being the optimum. If the temperature falls below 50° F (10° C) all feeding ceases, but the grubs seem to be able to survive a period of inactivity of months without dying, and can start feeding again as soon as the temperature rises. Dry heat at over 130° F (55° C) kill the grubs rapidly, and if prolonged, the unhatched eggs. In hot water, 30 seconds at 140° F (60° C) will destroy eggs and grubs, as will strong sunlight or ultraviolet light.

It is estimated that about 45 million pounds of wool are destroyed annually by clothes moths. In buildings, the greatest danger is to carpets and upholstery, and the insects are attracted to sheltered positions, underneath chairs or desks or in the lower portions of upholstered furniture, so the infestation may become quite heavy before anything is noticed. Regular and thorough cleaning is the greatest weapon against the moths. If a carpet is vacuumed regularly and occasionally shampooed, it need never be attacked. However, if grubs or moth holes are found, the carpet or furniture must be cleaned thoroughly and then treated with lindane or dieldrin. Carpets must be taken up and treated on both sides, and furniture treated similarly—the underside of a chair, although not wool, can sometimes harbor grubs.

Para-dichlorobenzene crystals can be used as a moth repellent; it is not lethal, however, and for the same amount of trouble an insecticide could be sprayed on.

## WOODWORM

The most common source of "worm" in lumber and furniture is the furniture beetle, *Anobium punctatum.* This insect lays 20 to 40 eggs in crevices in woodwork, and these develop into grubs in 3 to 4 weeks. The grubs are wood-borers, and live on the starches and sugars in the wood. For this reason they prefer the sapwood to the heartwood, though it must be admitted that they are not very selective feeders. Plywood and basketwork are particularly liable to attack. The boring goes on for a year or more, and then the grubs change into a chrysalis stage. In 2 to 3 weeks the chrysalis changes into an adult beetle, and this emerges from the wood, leaving the characteristic "flight hole" which is the best-known evidence of woodworm infestation. It should be understood from the life history of the creature, however, that the flight holes represent only the last stage of a long sequence of damage. While there are still very few flight holes, there may be hundreds of grubs eating the wood below the surface.

In the treatment of affected wood, first remove as much as possible of the fine powdered "sawdust" left by the grubs. This is to make the flight holes as accessible as possible to the insecticidal liquid. Specialized firms deal both with the insecticides and the application, and anyone faced with woodworm infestation would be well advised to call in such specialists.

# Index